ATLAS OF
Breast
Reconstruction

LUIS O. VASCONEZ, MD

Professor and Chief
Department of Surgery
Division of Plastic Surgery
The University of Alabama at Birmingham
Birmingham, Alabama, USA

MADELEINE LEJOUR, MD

Professor and Chairman
Department of Plastic Surgery
Brugmann University Hospital
Brussels, Belgium

MABEL GAMBOA-BOBADILLA, MD

Research Assistant Professor
Department of Surgery
Division of Plastic Surgery
The University of Alabama at Birmingham
Birmingham, Alabama, USA

Forewords by
Marshall Urist, MD
Aldo Piccolo, MD

With Original Illustrations by Alan Landau

J.B. LIPPINCOTT COMPANY • PHILADELPHIA
GOWER MEDICAL PUBLISHING • NEW YORK • LONDON

Distributed in USA and Canada by:
J.B. Lippincott Company
East Washington Square
Philadelphia, PA 19105 USA

Distributed in UK and Continental
Europe by:
Harper & Row Ltd
Middlesex House
34-42 Cleveland Street
London W1P 5FB UK

Distributed in Australia
and New Zealand by:
Harper & Row (Australia) Pty Ltd
P.O. Box 226
Artarmon, NSW 2064, Australia

Distributed in Southeast Asia,
Hong Kong, India, and Pakistan by:
Harper & Row Publishers (Asia) Pte Ltd
37 Jalan Pemimpin 02-01
Singapore 2057

Distributed in Japan by:
Igaku Shoin Ltd
Tokyo International
P.O. Box 5063
Tokyo, Japan

ISBN 0-397-44662-4

Library of Congress Cataloging-in-Publication Data

Vasconez, Luis O.
    Atlas of breast reconstruction / Luis O. Vasconez, Madeleine
Lejour, Mabel Gamboa-Bobadilla ; contributors, James C. Grotting,
Rama P. Mukherjee, Henry C. Vasconez ; with original illustrations
by Alan Landau.
        p.   cm.
    Includes bibliographical references.
    ISBN 0-397-44662-4
    1. Mammaplasty. 2. Musculoskeletal flaps. 3. Mammaplasty-
-Complications and sequelae. I. Lejour, Madeleine. II. Gamboa-
-Bobadilla, Mabel.   III. Title.
    [DNLM: 1. Breast—surgery—atlases. 2.Mastectomy—atlases.
3. Surgery, Plastic—methods—atlases. 4. Surgical Flaps—atlases.]
RD539.8.V37 1990
618.1'9059—dc20
DNLM/DLC
for Library of Congress   90-3911
                                                              CIP

British Library Cataloging-in-Publication Data

Vasconez, Luis O.
    Atlas of breast reconstruction.
    1. Women. Breasts. Plastic surgery
    I. Title II. Lejour, Madeleine III. Gamboa-Bobadilla,
    Mabel
    618. 19059

    ISBN 0-397-44662-4.

10 9 8 7 6 5 4 3 2 1   ·

Editor: Dimitry Popow
Art Director: Jill Feltham
Illustrator: Alan Landau
Designer: Paul E. Fennessy

Printed in Hong Kong by Imago

Contributors

James C. Grotting, MD
Associate Professor
Department of Surgery
Division of Plastic Surgery
The University of Alabama at Birmingham
Birmingham, Alabama

Rama P. Mukherjee, MD
Chief, Division of Plastic Surgery
Marshfield Clinic
Marshfield, Wisconsin

Henry C. Vasconez, MD
Assistant Professor
Division of Plastic Surgery
University of Kentucky
Lexington, Kentucky

Forewords

In 1880 surgeons were struggling with the problem of local and regional recurrence which followed soon after resection of a primary tumor from the breast. One of the goals of the standard radical mastectomy was accomplished by a comprehensive regional resection which lowered these recurrences to 10% or less. In large part because of its success rate, the radical mastectomy was accepted as the single method of treatment for all stages of breast cancer well into the 1960s. At present, we have a much improved understanding of the biology of cancer in general, and of the natural history of breast cancer in particular. This understanding has been gained through the efforts of thousands of patients and clinical investigators who have participated in prospective trials. These studies have conclusively shown that breast conservation therapy achieves the same local control rates and survival as mastectomy.

This remarkable transition over the past 20 years has created a new level of complexity which frustrates physicians and patients alike. More than half of the women with newly diagnosed breast cancer will qualify for conservation therapy, yet many will hesitate to choose this option because of uncertainties and misunderstandings about local recurrence, aesthetic appearance, irradiation, length of therapy, travel, and occasionally, cost. On the other hand, some women feel guilty when they choose mastectomy after being encouraged to conserve their breasts. It is now clear that there is no one best option for all patients.

Much of this anguish over decision making has been lessened by the alternative of breast reconstruction. The patient awakens from anesthesia with a breast that reduces the anxiety of physical loss, relieves her of the burden of an external prosthesis, and in some cases provides a better cosmetic result than an irradiated breast. This is not an ideal replacement, because the new breast is insensible and the opposite breast may require revision to create a satisfactory match. The use of autogenous tissue substantially lengthens the operation, prolongs convalescence, and may increase the risk of complications. Despite these disadvantages, increasing numbers of women are selecting reconstruction.

If patients are to be asked to make a truly informed decision about their treatment, they should be encouraged to have a consultation with both a radiation oncologist and a plastic surgeon. Talking with patients who have undergone each type of therapy is also often helpful. To counsel patients properly about the choices of treatment, the physician must have an in-depth understanding of each modality. Patients may have unrealistic expectations from reconstruction, just as with conservation therapy. The patient has the freedom to make her own decision, but the primary surgeon is still obligated to provide direction and recommendations.

The *Atlas of Breast Reconstruction* by Drs. Vasconez, Lejour, and Gamboa-Bobadilla is a comprehensive resource for all physicians who participate in breast cancer treatment. For the plastic surgeon, it is a magnificent description and teaching guide to complex procedures. For the oncologic surgeon, radiation therapist, and medical oncologist it is a complete and frank discussion of what can and cannot be accomplished with state-of-the-art techniques. Although refinements will undoubtedly occur, the fundamental principles outlined here will remain. It is hoped that many patients will benefit from the wisdom of this vast experience in breast reconstruction.

Marshall Urist, MD
Professor of Surgery
Chief, Section of Surgical Oncology
The University of Alabama at Birmingham

The expression of a patient who has undergone a mastectomy generally is either sad or hopeful. Sometimes a simple phrase or a few kind words are most welcome, giving the patient solace and comfort.

The picture changes when we see a patient who has undergone breast reconstruction, especially if it took place immediately after the mastectomy. In most cases, the patient projects self-confidence and a continued interest in life.

The addition of breast reconstruction to breast cancer therapy in most cases yields satisfactory results from both the human and the surgical standpoints.

Having started in the 1970s, breast reconstruction is a relatively new endeavor. The surgical results and techniques have improved to a usually satisfactory level, particularly with the introduction of sophisticated technology and greater choice of reconstructive procedures. In addition, the safety of prolonged operative time has increased thanks to advances in anesthesia. One can now state that, as long as an appropriate method is chosen, almost any postmastectomy defect can be reconstructed, and with predictable results in most cases.

Obviously, breast reconstruction cannot proceed until the pathology of the breast cancer and the variety of methods to treat it are clearly determined. The patient should receive clear and accurate information as to her choices, which may include conservative procedures with radiotherapy as well as mastectomy with immediate reconstruction. One should remember that most patients are undergoing adjuvant chemotherapy, and therefore no reconstructive procedure may interfere with such regimen. Fortunately, the multidisciplinary approach is now commonplace in most medical centers.

That reconstructive surgeons should be conscious of the limitations of their procedures and of their technical skills cannot be emphasized enough. It is the patient who suffers the consequences of a poorly planned or executed procedure.

The *Atlas of Breast Reconstruction* by Drs. Vasconez, Lejour, and Gamboa-Bodadilla demonstrates in a thoroughly illustrated fashion and with humbling honesty the different reconstructive procedures available to patients who have undergone mastectomy just before reconstruction or at some time in the past. I particularly liked their demonstration of the results "as they come," which included partial necrosis, asymmetry of the inframammary fold, and inadequate projection, which this book clearly teaches how to avoid, whenever possible.

I know the authors. I visited their clinics, I chatted with them at length on breast reconstruction—our favorite subject—and perhaps I have also influenced them in some of their ideas. What is more important, however, is their friendship, which I cherish. For me it is a matter of pride and personal satisfaction to introduce this book, which I think will be helpful not only to reconstructive surgeons but to all surgeons who treat breast diseases.

Aldo Piccolo, MD
Associate Professor, Plastic Surgery
Clinica Chirurgia Dell'Universita di Roma "La Spienza"
Rome, Italy

Preface

Breast reconstruction is now an established procedure, performed throughout the world with increasingly improved results. The entire area of breast cancer was thoroughly reevaluated in the 1960s and 1970s, mainly because the women who suffered from the disease pressed for a greater choice of treatment options. It was only natural for breast reconstruction to follow this trend and, as a result, to experience new safety and aesthetic demands.

Breast reconstruction is still an imperfect art. It prolongs operative time, takes multiple stages to accomplish a satisfactory result, and still has a significant percentage of complications. This situation should be unacceptable for an elective procedure aimed at aesthetic enhancement. We must strive for improvement. As our techniques develop, we venture to say that immediate reconstruction of the breast will become the rule for those patients who choose mastectomy as a treatment option for breast carcinoma.

This treatise compiles our experience with reconstruction of the breast. It is a subject that has involved us for the past 20 years, filling us with satisfaction as well as sadness—for we have felt dismay when reconstruction symmetry could not be achieved, and sadness as we faced the complications that sometimes ensued. These emotions have stimulated our desire to improve and to analyze all unsatisfactory outcomes.

As the reader will clearly see, our results indicate that we still have a way to go. We purposely have not attempted to show only our spectacular cases, but have in effect selected those average results which represent the majority of our patients. The term "average," however, has an unusually narrow range in our profession, with only a short distance separating the spectacular success from the spectacular failure. We have tried to indicate, step-by-step, important aspects of the different operative procedures, with an emphasis on the safe steps that should be taken to avoid unnecessary risks and complications.

The reader may observe that the book is unbalanced in that considerably more coverage is given to the autogenous method of breast reconstruction, particularly with the transverse rectus abdominis muscle (TRAM) flap. This method not only has yielded the best success, but also has allowed reconstruction in difficult cases (i.e., radiotherapy damage after tumorectomy) which otherwise would not have been amenable to reconstruction. We acknowledge that this is a bias in our present practice. We have not had the same type of satisfying results with the use of silicone implants and expanders as those we obtain with autogenous tissue. When we use implants or expanders, the number of operative procedures is usually greater (approximately three per patient) and the results are less reliable and predictable than those with autogenous tissue. It is possible that our opinion will change as new experience is gained with the more predictable textured or polyurethane-covered implants. In fact, as this is being written, we are using more textured or polyurethane-covered implants than plain silicone prostheses in immediate reconstructions.

We have attempted to include in this volume the most common problems encountered during breast reconstruction. The readers, depending on their experience, may differ on the procedures indicated in this book, which is quite understandable because there are many ways to accomplish the same objective. We have tried to indicate the principles and problems encountered, as well as the safeguards to be taken during a particular method of reconstruction. This volume should help the beginning as well as the more experienced reconstructive surgeon. The former will learn the steps taken in the reconstructive procedure while the latter will gain additional acumen—as well as the certitude that a procedure was well chosen and executed even when the outcome was less than perfect.

Luis O. Vasconez, MD
Madeleine Lejour, MD
Mabel Gamboa-Bobadilla, MD

Acknowledgments

To my wife and my daughters, who gave me constant support. To my residents, who taught me more about breast reconstruction than I ever contributed to them, and to my patients, who allowed me the privilege to operate on them and to try newer techniques.

Luis O. Vasconez, MD

To the past and present members of the plastic surgery teams. Not only did they take good care of the patients, but they also provided invaluable help in reviewing their files and improving their treatments.

Madeleine Lejour, MD

To my parents, my husband Ever, and my son Christopher, for their love, devotion, and encouragement.

Mabel Gamboa-Bobadilla, MD

Contents

INTRODUCTION

Principles of Breast Reconstruction	I.2
Symmetry	I.2
Creation and Location of the Inframammary Fold	I.4

CHAPTER 1   THE MASTECTOMY PROCEDURE

History	1.2
The Halsted Radical Mastectomy	1.3
The Modified Radical Mastectomy	1.7
The Auchincloss–Madden Technique	1.9
The Scanlon Technique	1.9
Breast Preserving Operations	1.10
Chemotherapy and Radiotherapy in Breast Cancer	1.13

CHAPTER 2   BREAST RECONSTRUCTION WITH IMPLANTS AND EXPANDERS

Simple Insertion of an Implant	2.2
Bilateral Reconstruction of the Breast with Insertion of Silicone Implants	2.9
Creation of the Inframammary Fold	2.10
Muscle Coverage of the Implant	2.10
Reconstruction with Skin Expanders	2.17
The Lower Thoracic Advancement Flap in Breast Reconstruction (Ryan–Pennisi Method)	2.21
Bilateral Reconstruction with Simple Placement of Implants in an Obese Patient	2.26

CHAPTER 3   BREAST RECONSTRUCTION WITH LATISSIMUS DORSI MYOCUTANEOUS FLAP

Principles	3.2
Surgical Technique	3.3
Reconstruction of Both Breasts with Bilateral Latissimus Dorsi Myocutaneous Flaps	3.14
Preoperative Planning	3.14
Surgical Technique	3.15
Revision of Breast Reconstruction with a Latissimus Dorsi Myocutaneous Flap	3.19

CHAPTER 4   BREAST RECONSTRUCTION WITH FLAPS

Lower Transverse Rectus Abdominis Muscle Flap and
    Abdominal Wall Closure   4.2
Selection of Patients   4.8
Variations Due to Abdominal Scars   4.32
Bilateral TRAM Flap Breast Reconstruction   4.39
Bilateral TRAM Flap Reconstruction—
    Mastectomy of the Contralateral Breast at Risk   4.43

CHAPTER 5   CONTRALATERAL UPPER RECTUS FLAP
               FOR BREAST RECONSTRUCTION

Indications   5.2
Surgical Technique   5.2

CHAPTER 6   IMMEDIATE POSTMASTECTOMY BREAST RECONSTRUCTION

Indications   6.2
Intraoperative Management   6.2
Methods   6.3
Complications   6.4

CHAPTER 7   PROCEDURES ON THE OPPOSITE BREAST

Preoperative Decisions   7.2
Mastopexy   7.3
Breast Reduction and Mastopexy   7.6
Breast Augmentation and Mastopexy   7.11
Reduction Mammaplasty   7.11
Breast Augmentation   7.16

CHAPTER 8   RECONSTRUCTION OF THE NIPPLE–AREOLA COMPLEX

Selection of Methods   8.2
Surgical Technique   8.3
The Skate Method   8.8

CHAPTER 9   SPECIAL PROBLEMS AND SECONDARY CORRECTIONS

Inframammary Crease   9.2
TRAM Flap with Percutaneous Re-Creation of the Inframammary Fold   9.3
Special Reconstruction Problems   9.4
Male Breast Carcinoma and Reconstruction   9.4
TRAM Flap After Latissimus Dorsi Muscle Failure   9.8
Congenital Breast Asymmetry   9.10
Poland's Anomaly   9.10
Severe Deformity   9.12
TRAM Flap to Correct Subcutaneous Mastectomy—Persistent Problems   9.14
Subclavicular (Hollow) Defect   9.16

CHAPTER 10   BREAST CARCINOMA: TREATMENT AND RECONSTRUCTION OF LOCAL RECURRENCES OR POSTRADIATION ULCERS

Local Recurrences   10.2
Postradiation Ulcers   10.2
Treatment   10.2
Postlumpectomy and Irradiation Defects   10.6

CHAPTER 11   SECONDARY BREAST RECONSTRUCTION ALTERNATIVES

TRAM Flap Reconstruction After Implant Complications   11.2
De-Epithelialized TRAM Flap for Autogenous Tissue Augmentation   11.4

CHAPTER 12   SUBCUTANEOUS MASTECTOMY AND RECONSTRUCTION

Surgical Technique   12.3
Precautions   12.6

CHAPTER 13   IMMEDIATE BREAST RECONSTRUCTION USING THE FREE TRAM FLAP
James C. Grotting, MD

Surgical Technique   13.2
Postoperative Management   13.7
Clinical Case   13.9

CHAPTER 14   COMPLICATIONS

Recurrent Carcinoma in the Reconstructed Breast   14.2
Partial Flap Necrosis—Flap Extended Beyond
    the Lower Midline Abdominal Scar   14.3
Complex Reconstruction for Silicone Injections of the Breast   14.4
Exposure of the Implant in Poland's Syndrome   14.7
Abdominal Hernia   14.8
A Double Fold of the Vascular Pedicle of the TRAM Flap   14.9
Conventional TRAM Flap with Microvascular Enhancement   14.10
Early Abdominal Reexploration   14.14

CHAPTER 15   POSTMASTECTOMY RECONSTRUCTION WITH IPSILATERAL UPPER RECTUS MYOCUTANEOUS FLAP
Rama P. Mukherjee, MD

Anatomic Considerations   15.2
Patient Selection   15.2
Patient Preparation and Surgical Technique   15.3
Complications   15.5
Reconstruction of the Nipple–Areola Complex   15.5
Operation on Opposite Breast   15.5

CHAPTER 16   POLYURETHANE-COVERED IMPLANTS AND PERMANENT TISSUE EXPANDERS FOR IMMEDIATE RECONSTRUCTION
Henry C. Vasconez, MD

Polyurethane-Covered Implants   16.2
Biologic Considerations   16.3
Clinical Differences of Smooth and Polyurethane (Textured) Implants   16.4
Clinical Experience with Implants and Autogenous Tissue   16.5
Permanent Tissue Expander (Becker Prosthesis)   16.8

INTRODUCTION

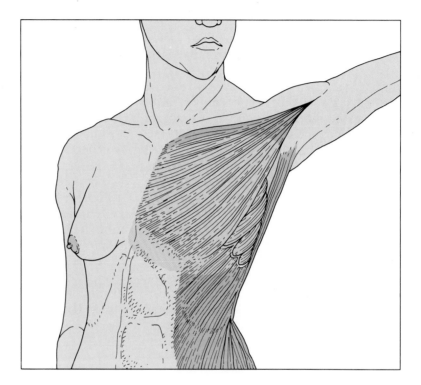

PRINCIPLES OF BREAST RECONSTRUCTION

The objective of breast reconstruction is to obtain symmetry with a normal breast and to do so using a safe and relatively simple procedure. Breast symmetry is more likely to result from simultaneous reconstruction of both breasts which have received similar mastectomies, using the same technique and resulting in similar scars. Symmetry is more difficult to achieve in a patient who has had dissimilar mastectomies, such as a modified radical on one side and a subcutaneous one on the opposite side.

Because reconstruction of a breast is an elective procedure, safety should be kept uppermost in the surgeon's mind. Whenever possible, autologous blood transfusions should be used. Simplicity is a worthwhile aim, but unfortunately not always achievable—particularly if reconstruction involves the use of autologous tissue and a transverse abdominal island flap. This procedure is not simple, but the aim should be to make it safe.

Symmetry

A reconstructed breast should match the breast on the opposite side. If bilateral reconstruction is performed, both breasts should have equal projection, and their inframammary creases should be at the same level. In most cases, symmetry is not achieved because of the incorrect placement of the inframammary crease. Other common problems are inadequate projection, and abnormal contour and ptosis of the newly reconstructed breast. With increasing clinical experience, we have learned to control and correct some of these failings.

Inframammary Line

The inframammary line represents the lower edge of breast tissue as it attaches to the chest wall. It is also determined by the lower edge of a capsule surrounding an implant or by the inferior edge of the transverse rectus abdominis muscle (TRAM) flap. Just as important, one can create an inframammary line by suturing the underlying subcutaneous tissue, or dermis, to the chest wall.

Although the inframammary crease can be easily delineated from the normal contralateral side, it is affected by the type of reconstructive procedure performed and subsequent biological factors of healing. For example, if a silicone implant is used, the ensuing capsular contracture is likely to bring up the inframammary crease. If the entire inframammary crease has been erased by inferior dissection during a mastectomy, the proper location of the inframammary line is lost. Consequently, when reconstructing a breast with a TRAM flap, a surgeon is likely to place the lower edge of the flap either too high or too low.

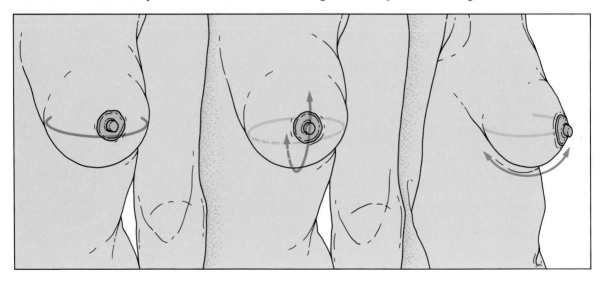

FIG. I.1

Projection

The breast is a three-dimensional structure, and on a patient who has undergone mastectomy, the curved surface has been turned into a flat one. Projection is determined by a curved, transverse line that begins at the anterior axillary line and extends toward the lateral border of the sternum. A round, youthful breast will have more projection than an atrophic, ptotic breast. A silicone implant or an expander is likely to give considerable projection—the limiting factor being the elasticity of the skin that lies between two fixed points, one positioned at the anterior axillary line, and the other at the lateral border of the sternum *(Fig. I.1)*.

In TRAM flap reconstruction, projection is obtained by coning the flap so that the umbilicus site is at 6 o'clock. Portions of zones I and II (see *Fig. 4.14* in Chapter 4) are coned *(Fig. I.2)*. If the flap is rotated differently (i.e., with a vertical placement), then the surgeon can achieve projection by de-epithelializing and tucking under zone III at the level of the anterior axillary line.

Tightness of the skin in the transverse diameter, from the sternum to the midaxillary line, precludes the use of larger implants or the burying of de-epithelialized tissue to obtain greater projection. However, one can increase the transverse dimension in the chest's skin by using a zigzag incision on the upper flap *(Fig. I.3)*, by using skin expanders that stretch the skin, or by using vertically placed skin, as is done in the latissimus dorsi method of reconstruction *(Fig. I.4)*.

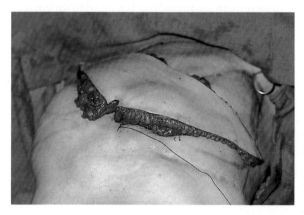

FIG. I.2

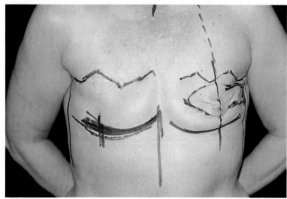

FIG. I.3

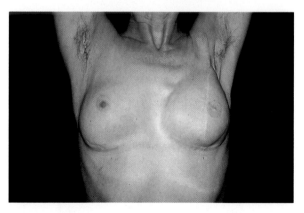

FIG. I.4

Ptosis

Ptosis is determined by the amount of breast tissue that usually droops below the inframammary line. To obtain ptosis, the inframammary line must be fixed securely; then the tissue of the reconstructed breast must be allowed to flow under this line and hang from it. We have not learned how to obtain ptosis with the use of silicone implants or expanders. However, we have been moderately successful in obtaining a semblance of ptosis by using autogenous tissue in breast reconstruction.

In short, the key to breast reconstruction is the creation of an inframammary line that is at the same level as the contralateral one. Ptosis will be observed against this fixed line. One can control projection, in turn, by coning the flap, zigzagging the upper flap incision, or adding tissue *(Fig. I.5)*.

Creation and Location of the Inframammary Fold

Creating or placing the inframammary fold at the proper level is not easy. If the inframammary fold has not been dissected out by the oncology surgeon, it can be used to place the lower edge of the TRAM flap. Hence, during immediate breast reconstruction with autogenous tissue, the surgeon should attempt to leave undisturbed at least a portion of the inframammary fold.

If an elective, unilateral breast reconstruction with autogenous tissue is to be performed, the surgeon should mark the inframammary line by using markings from the contralateral breast or by using the exterior markings of the removable prosthesis that the patient is using. If necessary, the line can be tattooed with methylene blue. The lower skin flap is then dissected down to (no more than 1 cm below) the tattooed line, which is where the lower edge of the TRAM flap eventually is placed.

Due to the muscle pedicle of the TRAM flap, the medial end of the inframammary line will not be well delineated at first. But the medial end will be re-created secondarily and percutaneously as described in Chapter 9. It is usually done at the same time as the nipple reconstruction.

When reconstructing the breast with an expander or implant, we believe that the inframammary fold needs to be created and fixed prior to the insertion of the prosthesis. In this case, the upper abdominal skin must be advanced up, as much as possible, so that enough skin is provided for the placement of the implant or expander. We suggest the creation of the inframammary crease as demonstrated in Chapter 9. When expanders or implants are used, however, the reconstructed inframammary crease should be fixed at least 2 to 4 cm below the contralateral one; this procedure allows for the capsular contracture that will occur.

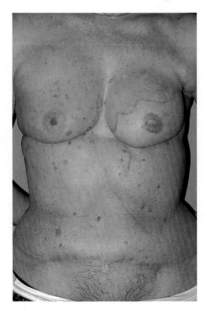

FIG. I.5

The principle of re-creating the inframammary fold was demonstrated by Lewis,[1] Pennisi,[2] and Ryan,[3] who were first to understand this development. Ryan realized that the weight of the implant, either filled with silicone or saline, pushes against this fixed line, stretches the skin, and in time gives a semblance of ptosis to the reconstructed breast. Similarly, when using an expander, Versaci and Balkovich[4] attempted to fix the inframammary crease internally and to use the extra expanded skin to provide ptosis.

When choosing expanders or the Becker-type implants, one should consider other adjunctive principles, such as covering the implants with as much muscle as possible and inflating them slowly, usually over a period of at least 2 months. In an effort to overcome problems of "recall," such as shrinkage of the expanded skin after replacement of the expander with a permanent implant, one should wait a prolonged period of time. It is not known how long this period should be; we recommend a minimal wait of 4 to 6 months.

The main focus in breast reconstruction is the fixation of the inframammary crease, regardless of the method used. In this atlas, the different techniques of breast reconstruction are described in detail.

REFERENCES

1. Lewis JR Jr: Use of a sliding flap from the abdomen to provide cover in breast reconstructions. *Plast Reconstr Surg 1979;64:491.*
2. Pennisi VR: Making a definite inframammary fold under a reconstructed breast. *Plast Reconstr Surg 1977;60:523.*
3. Ryan JJ: A lower thoracic advancement flap in breast reconstruction after mastectomy. *Plast Reconstr Surg 1982;70:153.*
4. Versaci AD, Balkovich ME: Tissue expansion, in Habal M (ed): *Advances in Plastic and Reconstructive Surgery, Volume 1.* Chicago, Year Book, 1984, 95–145.

CHAPTER·1

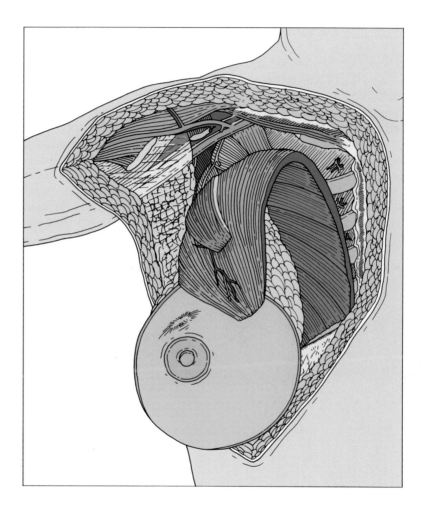

The Mastectomy
Procedure

HISTORY

Surgical treatment of carcinoma of the breast has been developed within the last century. As late as 1853, Sir James Paget of England, one of the foremost surgeons of his time, indicated that surgical extirpation of the breast was merely a palliative procedure. In 1867, Charles H. Moore, a surgeon at Middlesex Hospital, formulated his new principle of treatment of breast cancer that consisted of the removal of the entire breast and its axillary lymph nodes. In 1875, Richard von Volkmann added removal of the pectoral fascia with the breast and axillary lymph nodes. At the same time he introduced Lister's antiseptic methods, increasing the safety of such surgical procedures.

The final step in the evolution of the operation, known today as the radical mastectomy, was made in 1882 by William Stewart Halsted, an heroic figure in modern surgery at Johns Hopkins University. Although Halsted had received his medical education in New York, he had spent time in Germany and was aware of Volkmann's surgical ideas.

Halsted's first description of the operation, which he had performed in 13 cases of breast carcinoma, was published in 1891. He advanced the concept of a radical surgical attack upon carcinoma of the breast that included removal of a tumor with a margin of normal surrounding tissue. Halsted was one of the few surgeons of his day who had mastered the technique of skin grafting, which permitted him to remove as much tissue from a chest wall as he wished and to close the wound without tension. The concept of eradicating a tumor with a large amount of surrounding normal tissue and all regional lymphatics was extended to the dissection of the internal mammary chain by Jerome Urban in the 1950s.

Now, the trend in breast surgery is to return to smaller operations on the assumption that breast carcinoma is often a systemic disease. Local extirpation of a tumor is performed and is supplemented with adjuvant forms of therapy, such as radiotherapy, chemotherapy, or hormonal therapy. Thus, the modalities for treating carcinoma of the breast have come almost full circle.

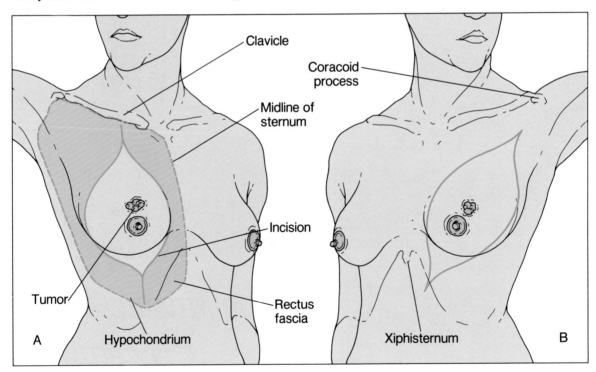

FIG. 1.1

THE HALSTED RADICAL MASTECTOMY

Surgical Technique

Dissection of the Skin Flap

Halsted's procedure for a radical mastectomy begins by drawing an ellipse or circle around the breast with the tumor near its center. Vertical extensions are then added above and below the circle. The superior extension must be high enough to give adequate access to the axilla. The lower vertical extension is carried straight downward over the hypochondrium *(Fig. 1.1.A)*. Modifications of the skin incisions have been devised as shown in

Fig. 1.1.B. The skin flaps are elevated just below the subdermal plexus at 2 to 3 mm in thickness *(Fig. 1.2)*. Raising skin flaps at this thickness is important to preserve the superficial plexus of vessels that ensure the viability of the overlying skin. Elevation of the skin flaps at the subdermal level, advocated by a decreasing number of surgeons, impairs the viability of the flaps.

Division of the Pectoralis Major Muscle from the Arm

Dissecting the skin flap laterally exposes the cephalic vein which separates the pectoralis major from the deltoid muscle. The cephalic vein is fol-

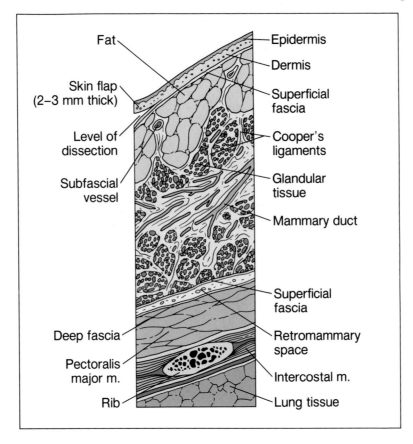

FIG. 1.2

lowed along the deltopectoral groove to the point where the pectoralis major muscle is attached to the humerus. The muscle is then cut across at a right angle to the direction of its fibers, preferably near its tendinous insertion. The division of the muscle insertion brings into view the deep pectoral fascia covering the structures of the axilla. Most surgeons spare the clavicular portion of the pectoralis major muscle to avoid an unsightly hollowness *(Fig. 1.3)*.

Dissection of the Pectoralis Major Muscle from the Clavicle

The pectoralis major muscle is dissected along the cephalic vein to the clavicle where it is separated from the deltoid. The thoracoacromial vessels and the lateral anterior thoracic nerve emerge from the deep pectoral fascia and are clamped, cut, and tied. The pectoralis major muscle is divided from the clavicle, cutting 1 cm below the lower edge of the clavicle. Again, most surgeons preserve the cla-

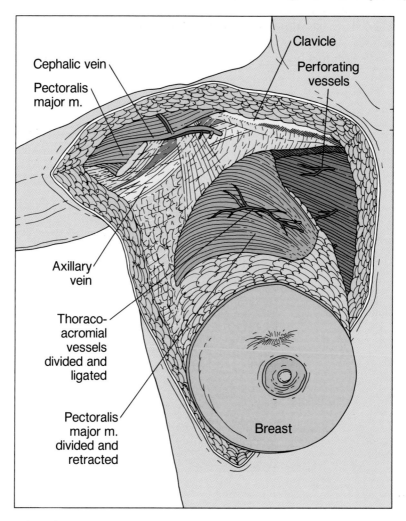

FIG. 1.3

THE MASTECTOMY PROCEDURE

vicular portion of the pectoralis major, which is easily done by blunt dissection.

Dissection of the Pectoralis Major Muscle from the Chest Wall

The pectoralis major is freed from its broad origin along the sternum, costal cartilages, and ribs. The dissection extends down to the fascia of the rectus abdominis and external oblique muscles *(Fig. 1.4)*. Most surgeons remove a portion of the anterior rectus sheath but care must be exercised to control the bleeding from the perforating vessels of the internal mammary artery, which emerge parasternally along the intercostal spaces.

Dissection of the Pectoralis Minor Muscle

The pectoralis minor muscle is divided 2 or 3 cm from its origin on the coracoid process. The thoracoacromial branch, which lies just lateral to the pectoralis minor muscle, has been previously divided. The muscle fibers are peeled from the third, fourth, and fifth ribs.

Dissection of the Axilla

As the breast and the pectoral muscles are dissected from the chest wall, they come to rest against the patient's side. The axilla is exposed at the cleft, which becomes a tetrahedral space, with the apex at the clavicle and the base at the pit of

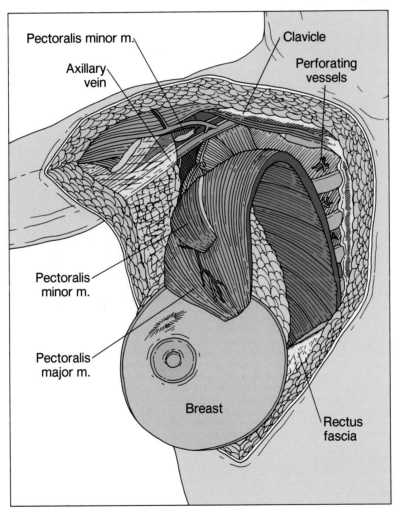

FIG. 1.4

the axilla. The three elongated triangular walls of this space are formed by the shoulder structures cephalically, the chest wall caudally, and the pectoral muscles ventrally.

The dissection of the axilla is begun by incising the deep pectoral fascia over the brachial plexus parallel with but slightly cephalad to the axillary vein. The ventral and caudal surfaces of the axillary vein are meticulously cleared from the level of the thoracoacromial vessels, medially, to the point where the vein crosses the white tendon of the latissimus dorsi muscle. All branches of the vein are isolated and divided between ligatures. The apex of the axilla is dissected by removing all the fat and areolar tissue of the axillary vein, medially, to the point at which it crosses beneath the subclavius muscle which is mobilized in the cleft between the

chest wall and the most medial portion of the axillary vein. The apex of the axilla contains the highest axillary lymph node and the lymphatic trunks.

The mass of tissue between the medial portion of the vein and the chest wall is dissected downward and outward off the surface of the subscapular muscle. The long thoracic nerve of Bell is left as the only structure crossing, in a longitudinal direction, the medial part of the axilla. This nerve, which innervates the serratus anterior muscle, is preserved because cutting it produces a deformity known as "winged scapula," as well as considerable shoulder pain that may last for months after surgery. The thoracodorsal vessels and thoracodorsal nerve supplying the latissimus dorsi muscle are sacrificed in most classical Halsted radical mas-

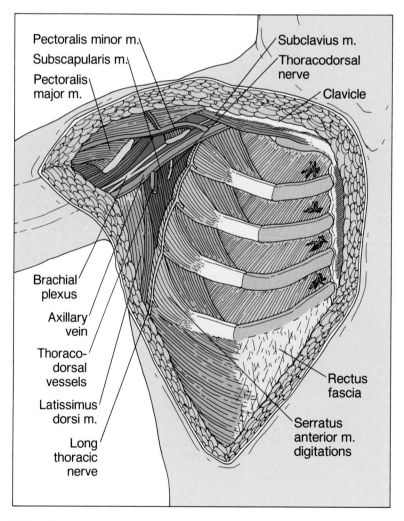

FIG. 1.5

THE MASTECTOMY PROCEDURE

tectomies. (One may still perform the latissimus dorsi method of breast reconstruction because of retrograde flow through the branch that supplies the serratus anterior muscle, but it is risky.) The dissection is completed by freeing the specimen from the medial edge of the latissimus dorsi muscle *(Fig. 1.5).*

Closure of the Wound

Skin flaps are replaced on the chest wall and sutured together without tension. Occasionally, the defect is covered with a skin graft. Suction catheters or drains are necessary, particularly along the region of the axilla.

THE MODIFIED RADICAL MASTECTOMY

In 1948, Patey and Dyson[22] devised an operative procedure that called for leaving the pectoralis major muscle intact while removing the breast, the pectoralis minor, and the axillary contents. These surgeons were influenced by the anatomical studies of Gray, which showed that while the skin was particularly rich in lymphatics, the pectoral fascia

was relatively free of lymphatic channels and, therefore, an unlikely route for the spread of cancer.

Surgical Technique

Opening

The incision is begun by marking out a circle of skin 5 cm clear of the palpable edge of the tumor. In every case, the nipple and areola are included, regardless of the location of the tumor. From this circle, extensions are made that are either transverse or ascending *(Fig. 1.6).*

Dissection of the Flaps

The flaps, 2 to 3 mm thick, are raised just below the subdermal vascular plexus. The medial flap is dissected to the midline of the chest, superior to a line that joins the sternal end of the clavicle with the lower edge of the insertion of the pectoralis major muscle into the humerus. Inferiorly, the flap is dissected below the breast into the hypochondrium and laterally, to the anterior edge of the latissimus dorsi muscle.

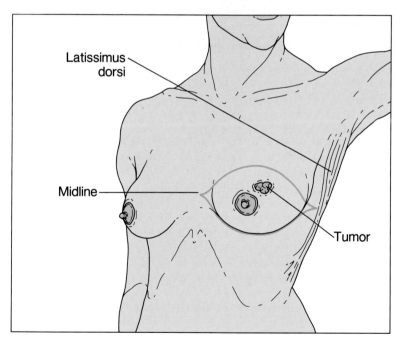

FIG. 1.6

Dissection of the Pectoralis Muscles

The breast tissue is freed from the pectoralis major muscle beginning medially and continuing laterally. It is better to include the pectoralis fascia and a few muscle fibers that may adhere to the back of the specimen. The arm is raised toward the ceiling to relax the pectoralis major muscle and a retractor is placed at the inferior edge of the muscle near the axilla to expose the origin of the pectoralis minor *(Fig. 1.7)*. The pectoral branch of the thoracoacromial artery and the lateral pectoral nerve are identified and preserved intact. If the medial pectoral nerve is divided, it will cause atrophy to the lateral portion of the pectoralis major. The origin of the pectoralis minor is divided from the coracoid process close to the bone. This exposes the apex of the axilla.

Dissection of the Axilla

The axillary vein is cleared exactly as is done in the Halsted technique. The thoracoacromial artery and vein are preserved, as is the thoracic nerve of Bell. The thoracodorsal nerve and vessels are also preserved.

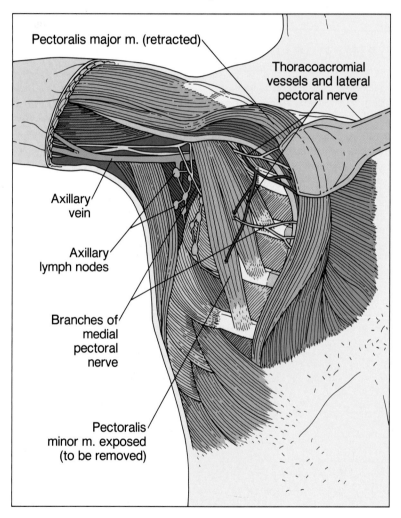

Pectoralis major m. (retracted)

Thoracoacromial vessels and lateral pectoral nerve

Axillary vein

Axillary lymph nodes

Branches of medial pectoral nerve

Pectoralis minor m. exposed (to be removed)

FIG. 1.7

Closure of the Wound

The specimen is removed and the wound is closed without tension, with or without the use of skin grafts. Suction catheters along the axilla are necessary.

Special Considerations

As determined by Scanlon,[25] the pectoral nerves need not be divided during the clearing of the axillary lymph nodes. This decision will preserve intact the function of the pectoralis major muscle. *Figure 1.7* shows the partially denervated pectoralis major following a Patey modified mastectomy procedure.

The advantages and disadvantages of the modified radical mastectomy are listed in *Table 1.1*. Several other versions of this procedure have been developed; two are described below.

The Auchincloss-Madden Technique

In 1963, Auchincloss[3] reviewed his findings and noted the extreme infrequency of involvement of apical lymph nodes in the absence of extensive lymph node metastasis. He suggested that breast cancer could be controlled by removing the breast and axillary nodes from the point opposite the approximate middle of the posterior surface of the pectoralis minor and laterally to the subscapular vessels. In 1972, Madden et al[19] described a similar operation. Preservation of the pectoralis minor and its nerve supply controls the tendency of the shoulder on the affected side to be elevated following either a modified or radical mastectomy. Injury to the medial pectoral nerve, which is inevitable if the pectoralis minor is divided, results in a varying amount of atrophy of the lateral and inferior parts of the pectoralis major muscle. Preservation of these nerves results in a more normal contour of the anterior axillary fold and of the chest wall.

The Scanlon Technique

Scanlon[24,25] modified the mastectomy by dividing the pectoralis minor muscle along its rib insertions. This action permits preservation of the pectoral nerves and provides good exposure of the axillary vessels. At the completion of the axillary

Table 1.1
The Modified Radical Mastectomy

ADVANTAGES	DISADVANTAGES
Preserves the pectoralis major muscle	Longer operative time
Exposes the pectoralis minor muscle, which is the key to the axilla. By either removing or dividing the muscle, the axilla can be cleared of fat and lymph nodes, with virtually the same efficiency as in the Halsted operation	The axilla is not cleaned as well as in the classical technique, particularly the interpectoral nodes of Rotter. These nodes lie around the pectoral branch of the thoracoacromial artery and the lateral pectoral nerve, both of which must be preserved intact if the pectoralis major muscle is to function
Preserves the thoracodorsal vessels and nerves	The arm on the operated side is slower to regain full movement because of the bruising that the pectoralis major muscle receives when it is denuded of all its fascia, as well as from the trauma of retraction. The return of full movement of the arm is slower if the pectoralis fascia is removed

dissection, the pectoralis major muscle is reattached to its remnants. Again, this procedure is emphasized because it preserves the medial and the lateral pectoral nerves, which are usually transected if the pectoralis minor muscle is divided from the coracoid process and retracted medially *(Fig. 1.8)*.

BREAST PRESERVING OPERATIONS

Breast Conservation Procedures

Conservation procedures for the management of breast cancer were advocated as early as 1928 by Keynes,[16] who presented the results of 42 patients with breast cancer treated with radium needles, with or without excisional biopsy. Since that time, multiple publications have reported on the use of local excision with a variety of radiotherapeutic techniques that allow local control of the primary cancer. Breast preserving procedures are usually appropriate only for the treatment of early breast cancer and in very select patients.

The contraindications to breast conservation procedures are diagrammed in *Figure 1.9.*

Size of the Primary Lesion

If the primary lesion is large in relation to the size of the breast, local excision would result in an unacceptable aesthetic result. Quadrantectomy alone should not be offered to women with tumors of 2 cm or larger because of the higher incidence of in-

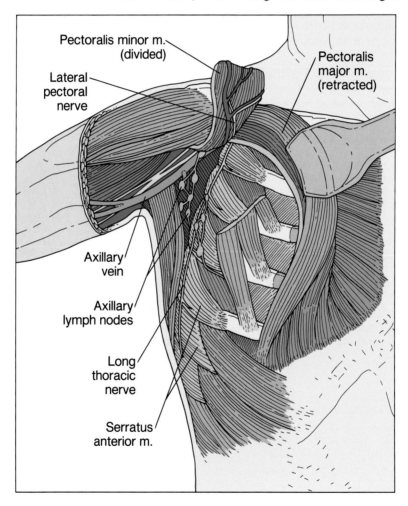

FIG. 1.8

vasive multicentric cancers. Initially, it is probably appropriate to limit this treatment to women with tumors of 2 cm or less in size.

Location of the Primary Lesion

Tumors located under the nipple are not amenable to local resection when their removal will sacrifice the nipple and areolar complex. One should note that 25 to 30% of patients have cancer involving the nipple,[17,23] and that nipple invasion is more frequent when the tumor is under the areola. Lagios et al[17] found 34% involvement of the nipple/areola when the tumor was within a 2.5-cm radius from the nipple. This would include most tumors that extend underneath the areola. When the primary tumor was 2.6 cm or further from the base of the nipple (not subareolar), only 14% of the patients had nipple invasion.

Multicentricity

Breast cancer is multicentric. After excision of the primary breast cancer, 21 to 31% of the women have another focus of cancer in another quadrant of the breast.[17,18,21] Multicentric invasive cancer is more frequently associated with large tumors. According to Lesser and colleagues,[18] T_1 tumors were

found to be associated with 7% multicentric invasive cancer, whereas primary tumors greater than 4 cm in diameter were associated with 30% invasive multicentric cancers. Multicentric cancers are encountered more frequently when the primary tumor is an infiltrating lobular carcinoma or infiltrating ductal carcinoma.

Margins of the Primary Lesion

If the primary lesion shows a diffuse or extensive *in situ* component, incomplete excision of the tumor or positive resection margins are associated with treatment failure. Mastectomy is advised in these instances.

Positive Nodes

Patients with clinically positive lymph nodes should also be excluded from treatment with quadrantectomy alone. Even in patients who are to undergo breast preserving operations, excisions and resections of the tumor, as well as an axillary dissection for staging, are performed.

Undifferentiated Carcinoma

Patients with undifferentiated carcinoma are best treated by mastectomy.

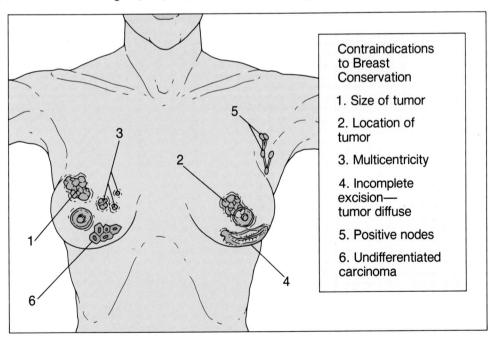

Contraindications to Breast Conservation

1. Size of tumor

2. Location of tumor

3. Multicentricity

4. Incomplete excision— tumor diffuse

5. Positive nodes

6. Undifferentiated carcinoma

FIG. 1.9

Excision of the Primary Lesion

Three types of local resection of primary lesions may be undertaken: excisional biopsy, wide local excision or tylectomy, and segmental mastectomy or quadrantectomy. In excisional biopsy, the primary cancer is removed with only a small rim of what grossly appears to be normal breast tissue *(Fig. 1.10.A)*. In wide local excision or tylectomy, a 1- to 2-cm margin of apparently normal breast tissue is removed from around the primary lesion with an ellipse of overlying skin *(Fig. 1.10.B)*. For the segmental mastectomy or quadrantectomy, approximately one quarter of the breast substance surrounding the primary lesion is removed.

Deformity of the breast is more likely to occur with this last option, especially if the lesion is in the upper, inner quadrant of the breast. When the primary tumor is in the upper, outer quadrant adjacent to the axilla, one can make a single incision to include removal of the primary tumor in continuity with the axillary dissection *(Fig. 1.10.C)*. When the primary tumor is in another quadrant of the breast, two separate incisions are made.

The skin incision should be oriented with respect for Langer's lines; radial incisions are avoided. Use of electrocautery is avoided during resection of the tumor to avoid denaturation of the steroid receptor protein.

Once excised, the specimen is available for histologic examination and for estrogen and progesterone receptor analysis. Frozen sections of all grossly suspicious margins should be performed.

Patients who have an excisional biopsy of the primary lesion fare better than those diagnosed by aspiration or by needle or drill biopsy and who are treated by radical radiotherapy only.[4]

Axillary Dissection

Axillary dissection may be achieved in three ways: blind axillary sampling, open axillary node dissection, and total axillary clearance *(Fig. 1.11)*.

Blind Axillary Sampling

In this procedure, a small transverse incision is made between the anterior and posterior axillary folds, giving access limited to the lower portion of the axilla. The axillary vein and the nerves to the serratus anterior and latissimus dorsi muscles are not exposed. Blind sampling is not recommended for routine use because the number of nodes re-

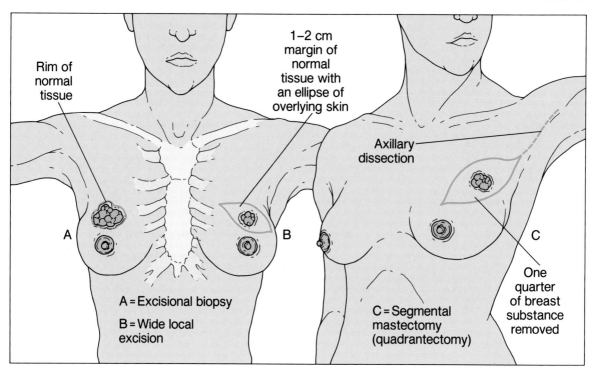

Rim of normal tissue

1–2 cm margin of normal tissue with an ellipse of overlying skin

Axillary dissection

A

B

C

One quarter of breast substance removed

A = Excisional biopsy

B = Wide local excision

C = Segmental mastectomy (quadrantectomy)

FIG. 1.10

moved is unlikely to be sufficient for adequate assessment of axillary node metastasis. Therefore, pathologic staging on which subsequent adjuvant therapy is determined may be inaccurate.

Open Axillary Node Dissection

Adequate exposure of the axillary vein and nerves to the serratus anterior and latissimus dorsi muscles can be achieved with this technique. All level I and some level II nodes can be removed.

Total Axillary Clearance

A complete dissection and removal of the axillary contents can be achieved for all three levels of the axilla, including the apex or level III nodes. The pectoralis minor muscle must be either transected or resected to accomplish the procedure. Total axillary clearance obviates the need to irradiate the axilla and is most valuable for pathologic staging.

CHEMOTHERAPY AND RADIOTHERAPY IN BREAST CANCER

Chemotherapy

Two types of treatment for potentially curable breast carcinoma include neoadjuvant chemotherapy and adjuvant chemotherapy.

Neoadjuvant Chemotherapy

This preoperative treatment was introduced by Frei and Canellos.[10] It is defined as treatment in one of three ways: (a) given at the earliest possible time in the tumor's natural history; (b) given before the definitive local/regional treatment; and (c) consisting of the most effective treatment regimen. The main rationale for neoadjuvant treatment is the assurance of the lowest possible systemic tumor cell burden at the time of the definitive

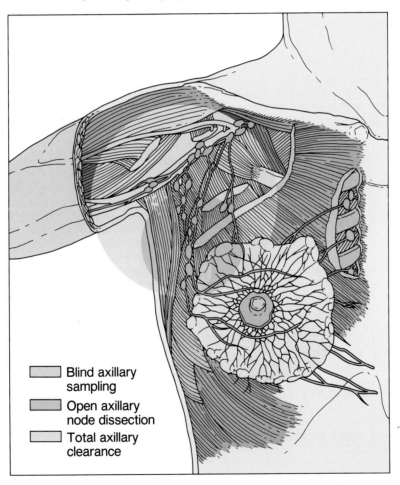

Blind axillary sampling

Open axillary node dissection

Total axillary clearance

FIG. 1.11

local/regional treatment. Chemotherapy administered before surgery may be more effective in controlling the spread or implantation of tumor cells which may be shed during surgery.

Adjuvant Chemotherapy

Studies by Fisher,[7] Bonadonna,[5] and their co-workers have offered strong evidence that patients with positive nodes who receive chemotherapy after mastectomy have prolonged survival without recurrence, as compared with patients treated by mastectomy alone. These results have been confirmed by the National Surgical Adjuvant Breast Project. Presently, most patients who are pre-menopausal with positive lymph nodes are submitted to a 6-month course of chemotherapy that includes cyclophosphamide methotrexate and 5-fluorouracil. The disease-free interval and overall survival advantages are quite clear in the treated

patients, and this chemotherapy may also be helpful for postmenopausal women. Recent findings indicate that adjuvant chemotherapy is also advisable for some premenopausal women with negative axillary nodes.

Radiotherapy

The role of radiotherapy in the treatment of breast cancer falls into three general categories: postoperative radiotherapy, radiotherapy following limited surgery, and radiotherapy for palliation in breast carcinoma.

Postoperative Radiotherapy

Postoperative radiotherapy decreases the incidence of local and regional recurrence through the control of residual subclinical disease *(Fig. 1.12)*. This is particularly important for patients in

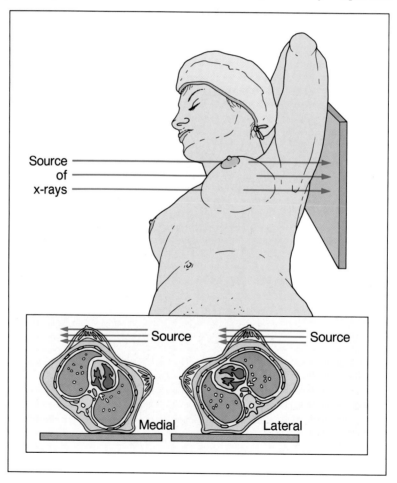

FIG. 1.12

THE MASTECTOMY PROCEDURE

whom the surgical removal has been inadequate or the deep margins or the resection showed tumor on pathologic examination. The option also improves the survival rate if metastatic dissemination can originate from local residual deposits, particularly those located in regional lymph nodes.

The radiation dosage required to control residual disease is 4,500 to 5,000 rads. The field to be irradiated depends on the type of surgery that has been performed. After mastectomy with axillary dissection, the irradiation of the axilla is not necessary because recurrences following proper axillary dissection are almost nonexistent. For patients who have had tumors situated in the central or inner quadrants of the breast with axillary metastasis, prophylactic radiation to the parasternal region is recommended.

Presently, adjuvant chemotherapy may be indicated when the axillary lymph nodes are involved, although chemotherapy and radiotherapy, given simultaneously, are not well tolerated. Patients, however, will tolerate hormonal therapy in the form of estrogen antagonists, given simultaneously with radiation therapy.

Radiotherapy Following Limited Surgery

As part of the informed consent, patients are offered the alternative of undergoing a lumpectomy and adjuvant radiation therapy as treatment for stage I breast carcinoma. The patient has to undergo a lumpectomy or quadrantectomy as well as an axillary dissection, either as a sampling or a full procedure for staging. Patients who make this choice are usually younger women with a strong desire to preserve the breast, who live longer and need longer follow-up treatment.

Presently, patients undergoing this breast conserving therapy are those with small tumors and clinically negative axillary lymph nodes. If, during the course of the lumpectomy or quadrantectomy, a tumor is noted at the margins or the tumor is multicentric, a modified mastectomy is advisable.

Early studies of this approach indicate survival as well as local recurrence rates comparable to those of modified mastectomy alone. This was demonstrated in the series by Veronesi et al,[27] who performed quadrantectomies as well as adjuvant radiotherapies. Series with longer follow-up, however, are beginning to show an increasing incidence of local recurrence in the range of 10 to 15%, particularly after 10 years. These results ap-

proximate the incidence of local recurrence following simple mastectomy alone for these early cancers. Thus, it appears that the lumpectomy and radiation therapy may delay the appearance of a local recurrence but it is still unclear whether the treated area is sterilized forever.

Radiotherapy for Palliation

Radiotherapy is invaluable for local control of inoperable breast carcinoma, particularly the ulcerated type. Preoperative radiotherapy is performed and may be followed by a palliated type of mastectomy to simplify the management of the wound.

Plastic surgeons see an increasing incidence of lymphedema of the arm among patients who have undergone axillary dissection as well as postoperative irradiation. The combination of the two modalities increases the incidence of lymphedema that can be expected from either modality alone.

Effect of Radiotherapy on Survival

The effect of radiation on survival is highly controversial and has been subjected to cooperative studies by the National Surgical Adjuvant Breast Project under the direction of Fisher et al[8,9] in 34 different clinics in the United States and Canada. During the initial studies, which ran from 1971 through 1974, women with operable breast carcinoma were also treated by radiation. The results were reported in 1977 after an average follow-up of 36 months. The initial report showed no difference in the survival between the patients who received radiotherapy and those who did not.

These findings were corroborated by subsequent studies. One report by Fisher et al in the *New England Journal of Medicine*[9] (1985) gives the 10-year survival rate for 1,665 eligible patients who were randomly assigned to treatment by radical mastectomy; mastectomy supplemented by radiation of the chest wall, the axilla and the internal mammary region; or mastectomy only for stage A patients (comparable with the TNM system at stage I). After 10 years there was no difference in the survival of patients in any of the three groups.

Other series, such as McWhirter's[20] or Kaae and Johansen's[15] reports of 10-year survival rates for mastectomy followed by radiation, as well as the longer follow-up of Fisher's series of clinical stage A cases,[9] show no advantage of added radiotherapy in the survival of patients undergoing breast cancer surgery.

In avoiding axillary recurrence, radical mastectomy is, however, much more effective than irradiation. Haagensen[13] showed no axillary recurrence in clinical stage A cases and only 1% in stage B cases. Kaae and Johansen[14] showed 8% in stage A cases and 18% in stage B cases in which the axilla was irradiated.

Another important finding was the superiority of the radical mastectomy performed by Haagensen as compared with a simple mastectomy supplemented by irradiation in preventing local recurrences of the chest wall. Haagensen showed only 3.7% of local recurrences within 10 years, while Kaae and Johansen found 10% of chest wall recurrence after simple mastectomy supplemented by irradiation.

Accepted Guidelines for Radiation Therapy

For patients who have had a local tumor excision or partial mastectomy without an axillary dissection, the entire breast, axilla, internal mammary and supraclavicular lymph nodes should be irradiated. The lymph node areas are usually given 4,500 to 5,000 rads over a 5-week period. Palpable axillary lymph nodes should receive an additional dose of about 1,000 rads per week.

Patients with a tumor in the outer quadrant and who show negative axillary lymph nodes need radiotherapy only to the breast itself. For patients who have an inner-quadrant lesion and negative axilla, the breast and internal mammary chain should be treated. When only an axillary sampling is performed and the nodes prove positive, radiation therapy should be given to the breast as well as to the regional lymph node areas.

When the axillary dissection removes the nodes at levels I and II, the apex of the axilla needs to be irradiated. In those patients who have had a complete dissection of nodes at levels I, II, and III, it is not necessary to irradiate the axilla. Adjuvant chemotherapy or hormonal therapy should be considered for patients with positive axillary lymph nodes. In all these patients, estrogen and progesterone receptors should be assayed on the excised tumor.

Limitations of Radiotherapy

Radiotherapy is ineffective in the management of preinvasive breast cancer, either intraductal or lobular carcinoma in situ, presumably because the biology of preinvasive breast cancer more closely approximates that of normal tissue. In his study of early breast cancer treated with radiotherapy, Harris et al[11] found that intraductal carcinoma was associated with a 5-year local recurrence of 39%.

Radiotherapy is inferior to adequate surgery for local control of large breast cancer. In the experience of the Foundation Curie,[6] 60% of patients with tumors larger than 3 cm required subsequent salvage surgery for either immediate or subsequent local failure. At the Marseilles Cancer Institute,[1] local failure was 10.5% for stage I, 25% for stage II, and 34% for patients not treated by prior surgical excision. About half of those failures are salvageable by mastectomy.

Radiotherapy is also inferior to surgery in preventing local and distant recurrence for larger breast cancers. A prospective randomized study from Guy's Hospital[2] compared radical mastectomy with wide local excision and radiotherapy. Both local recurrence and 10-year survival were quite similar for patients with stage I disease. For stage II patients, however, local control and survival were markedly inferior for the patients treated by wide excision and radiotherapy.

Radiotherapy requires long and frequent follow-up of patients. After a radical mastectomy, local recurrence appears most frequently in the first 2 or 3 years following treatment. After radiotherapy, local recurrence occurs at a constant rate of about 2% per year over at least 15 years, as found in the collective series of Harris et al.[12]

Local excision and radiotherapy offer no advantage over radical mastectomy in terms of postoperative physical or emotional problems. Schain et al[26] conducted a careful analysis of physical and psychosocial sequelae in patients randomized to either mastectomy or wide, local excision, axillary dissection, and radiotherapy. The only significant differences found in the numerous factors examined were better body image and more frequent shoulder stiffness in patients with intact breasts.

REFERENCES

1. Amalric R, Santamaria F, Robert F, et al: Radiation therapy with or without primary limited surgery for operable breast cancer: a 20-year experience at the Marseilles Cancer Institute. *Cancer 1982; 49:30.*
2. Atkins H, Hayward JL, Klugman DJ, et al:

Treatment of early carcinoma of breast. *Br Med J 1972; 2:423.*

3. Auchincloss H: Significance of location and number of axillary metastases in carcinoma of the breast. *Ann Surg 1963; 158:37.*

4. Bataini JP, Picco C, Martin M, et al: Relation between time-dose and local control of operable breast cancer treated by tumorectomy and radiotherapy or by radical radiotherapy alone. *Cancer 1978; 42:2059.*

5. Bonadonna G, Brusamolino E, Valagussa P, et al: Combination chemotherapy as an adjuvant treatment in operable breast cancer. *N Engl J Med 1976; 249:405.*

6. Calle R, Pilleron JP, Schlienger P, et al: Conservative management of operable breast cancer. Ten years experience at the Foundation Curie. *Cancer 1978; 42:2045.*

7. Fisher B, Carbone P, Economou SG, et al: l-phenylalanine mustard (L-PAM) in the management of primary breast cancer. A report of early findings. *N Engl J Med 1975; 292:117.*

8. Fisher B, Montague E, Redmond C, et al: Comparison of radical mastectomy with alternative treatments for primary breast cancer. *Cancer 1977; 39:2827.*

9. Fisher B, Redmond C, Fisher ER, et al: Ten-year results of a randomized clinical trial comparing radical mastectomy and total mastectomy with or without radiation. *N Engl J Med 1985; 312:674.*

10. Frei E III, Canellos GP: Dose: a critical factor in cancer chemotherapy. *Am J Med 1980; 69:585.*

11. Harris JR, Connolly JL, Schnitt SJ, et al: Clinical-pathologic study of early breast cancer treated by primary radiation therapy. *J Clin Oncol 1983; 1:184.*

12. Harris JR, Recht A, Amalric R, et al: Time course and prognosis of local recurrence following primary radiation therapy for early breast cancer. *J Clin Oncol 1984; 2:37.*

13. Haagensen CD, Bodian C: A personal experience with Halsted's radical mastectomy. *Ann Surg 1984; 199(2):143.*

14. Kaae S, Johansen H: Simple mastectomy plus postoperative irradiation by the method of McWhirter for mammary carcinoma. *Ann Surg 1969; 170:895.*

15. Kaae S, Johansen H: Does simple mastectomy followed by irradiation offer survival comparable to radical procedures? *Int J Rad Oncol Biol Phys 1977; 2:1163.*

16. Keynes G: Radium treatment of primary carcinoma of the breast. *Lancet 1928; 2:108.*

17. Lagios MD, Gates EA, Westdahl PR, et al: A guide to the frequency of nipple involvement in breast cancer. A study of 149 consecutive mastectomies using a serial subgross and correlated radiographic technique. *Am J Surg 1979; 138:135.*

18. Lesser ML, Rosen PP, Kinne DW: Multicentricity and bilaterality in invasive breast carcinoma. *Surgery 1982; 91:234.*

19. Madden JL, Kandalaft S, Bourque RA: Modified radical mastectomy. *Ann Surg 1972; 175:624.*

20. McWhirter R: Cancer of the breast. Symposium sur le Sein, Strasbourge. *J Radiol 1966; 48:768.*

21. Morgenstern L, Kaufman PA, Friedman NB: The case against tylectomy for carcinoma of the breast. *Am J Surg 1975; 130:251.*

22. Patey DH, Dyson WH: The prognosis of carcinoma of the breast in relation to the type of operation performed. *Br J Cancer 1948; 2:7.*

23. Quinn RH, Barlow JF: Involvement of the nipple and areola by carcinoma of the breast. *Arch Surg 1981; 116:1139.*

24. Scanlon EF, Caprini JA: Modified radical mastectomy. *Cancer 1975; 35:710*

25. Scanlon EF: The importance of the anterior thoracic nerves in modified radical mastectomy. *Surg Gyn Obstet 1981; 152:789.*

26. Schain W, Edwards BK, Gorell RC, et al: Psychosocial and physical outcome of primary breast cancer therapy: mastectomy vs excisional biopsy and irradiation. *Breast Cancer Res Treat 1983; 3:377.*

27. Veronesi U, Saccozzi R, Del Vecchio M, et al: Comparing radical mastectomy with quadrantectomy, axillary dissection and radiotherapy in patients with small cancers of the breast. *N Engl J Med 1981; 305:6.*

CHAPTER·2

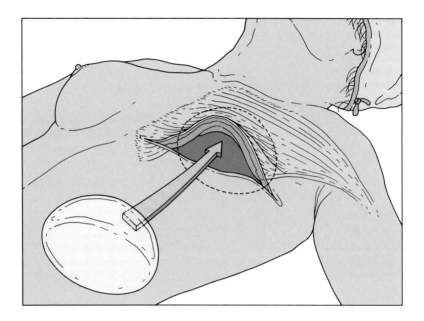

Breast Reconstruction with Implants and Expanders

SIMPLE INSERTION OF AN IMPLANT

The ideal candidate for a silicone implant is the patient who is neither thin nor obese, has a firm, rounded, and small opposite breast, a horizontal mastectomy scar with normal surrounding skin, and a well-preserved pectoralis muscle *(Fig. 2.1)*. A prosthesis should not be implanted under tight, thin, or irradiated skin, even if it is placed under the pectoralis muscle *(Fig. 2.2);* for the implantation would result in an unpleasant, painful capsular contracture, and it may lead to other more severe consequences, such as ulceration of the skin and extrusion of the implant.

Between these extremes, many cases are suitable for simple implantation, provided that a reconstructed breast of moderate size is acceptable to the patient. Sometimes, the patient who is offered a more sophisticated method of reconstruction prefers a simpler method with minimal hospitalization and disability, even if the result will be less perfect. Consideration of the patient's wish when one selects the method of reconstruction is more important today than it was several years ago, when fewer techniques were available. Many simple implantations have been performed in patients who were perfect candidates for TRAM flaps, for instance, but who did not desire such an extensive procedure. Implantations have been performed in other patients whose local condition might have been more suitable for a flap method of reconstruction, but they presented contraindications, such as poor general health, short life expectancy, or smoking habits.

About 30% of our patients choose simple implantation as a means of reconstructing the missing volume. In more than 80% of the cases, the other breast must be corrected for symmetry. This is done during the first procedure because it allows an additional correction in the breast's shape when the second stage of reconstruction takes place (areola-nipple reconstruction, if indicated.

The volume of the implant should be selected according to the patient's build and not the size of her other breast. In cases of moderate skin tension or thinness, it is safe to choose an implant somewhat smaller than ideal. Consequently, the implant is introduced first, before adjusting the opposite breast to the reconstructed side, unless the opposite breast has an adequate volume and requires only a mastopexy or a small implant to correct minimal ptosis.

Surgical Technique

It is advisable to place the implant through the mastectomy scar, rather than through a new incision *(Fig. 2.3.A, B)*. The mastectomy scar is incised 5 or 6 cm beginning at the level of the anterior axillary fold. The border of the pectoralis

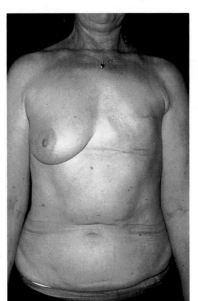

FIG. 2.1

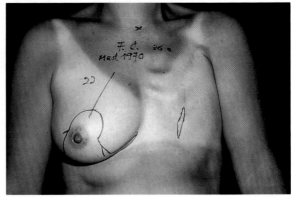

FIG. 2.2

muscle must be identified and the muscle lifted by blunt dissection. This is best done first by finger dissection with both hands, using the index and middle fingers of one hand to lift the muscle and skin while using the index finger of the other hand to dissect bluntly in all directions, detaching the lower and medial fibers of the pectoralis muscle *(Fig. 2.4)*. Dissection with long scissors is then continued caudally, under the serratus muscle, the external oblique muscles, and the fascia of the rectus muscle. Sometimes the dissection is subcutaneous and over the rectus fascia.

Submuscular dissection is sometimes impossible to do without tearing some muscle and fascia. This produces more bleeding and may create a tight coverage for the implant, which will be pushed up-

ward. On the other hand, a subcutaneous dissection may be made wider (we usually extend it to the upper part of the abdomen). This creates a large pocket for the implant, which will be covered by more skin with minimal tension. Hemostasis of a large pocket through a small incision is not easy. Bleeding may occur due to the division of medial or lateral intercostal perforators. Dissection in this region should therefore be done carefully, and as bluntly as possible. It may, however, be necessary to cut some adherences to the medial part of the mastectomy scar with scissors, but this rarely produces brisk bleeding.

If bleeding occurs, the whole dissected area (from the clavicle to the upper abdomen and from the axillary line to the midline) must be packed

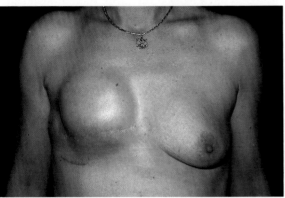

FIG. 2.3.A

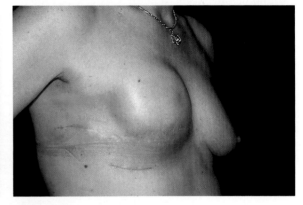

FIG. 2.3.B

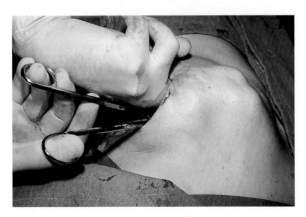

FIG. 2.4

temporarily and bleeding points cauterized by segmental visualization. The cavity is then rinsed with a dilute solution of Betadine, the patient is given intravenous antibiotics, and the implant is introduced carefully so that it is not torn *(Fig. 2.5)*.

It is important to ensure that no adherence remains in the pocket. The breast contour should not show any irregularity when the implant is pushed in all directions. If this happens, the implant should be taken out and the dissection completed.

Choosing the volume of the implant is difficult. We sometimes use an expansion prosthesis, and fill it until the volume seems adequate. We then replace it by an implant of the same size. During this procedure, a suction drain is placed in the wound before closing it in three layers, and the patient is given perioperative antibiotics. If the opposite breast requires correction, it is done during the same operation.

Postoperative Care

For the first week, the dressing holds the implant in a low and medial position. From the second day on, the patient is encouraged to massage her breast by pushing the implant downward, laterally, and medially several times a day. This activity maintains a wide pocket and may reduce the risk of capsular contracture and hardness of the breast. However, in most patients the implant fits tightly in the pocket, and massage is difficult or impossible.

The drain is left in place for 1 to 3 days. We have observed that the wound oozes for a longer period of time in patients who have had irradiation in the mastectomy region. The capsular contracture seems related to the oozing duration. If the drain must be left in place for more than 1 week, it is highly probable that a strong capsular contracture will develop in the following weeks.

The objective of the initial procedure is to

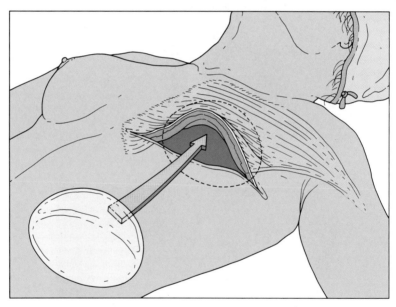

FIG. 2.5

achieve symmetry of volume and shape. This permits the second operation—the nipple-areolar reconstruction—to be a small, ambulatory procedure done under local anesthesia. It is not easy, however, to obtain good symmetry of shape and volume with one operation, as the reconstructed breast is rather flat after introduction of the implant *(Fig. 2.6)*. It will progressively take shape, volume, and position by the ensuing capsular contracture.

During the first week after surgery, the spontaneous upward displacement of the implant may be partly controlled by the dressing. If the breast tends to be too high, a bandage is wrapped under the axillae to push it down. On the contrary, if the implant remains too low, the patient is encouraged to wear a brassiere to keep it higher. After 3 or 4 weeks, these maneuvers are no longer useful, as the capsule is formed and the structure becomes less influenced by pressure. The patient is asked to massage her breast every day, but there is no proof that this is effective, as wound contracture is sometimes much stronger than any external force. A tight capsular contracture will require an open capsulotomy, which may be accompanied by an implant replacement if the volume is still unsatisfactory.

Capsular contracture is a phenomenon over which surgeons have little control. It has the advantage of shaping the breast, but also the disadvantage of sometimes displacing and distorting it. This is why it is impossible to predict exactly the shape and volume of the breast reconstructed with an implant. In our experience, more than 50% of the cases require a correction of volume, shape, or both at the time of areola reconstruction.

On the whole, placement of an implant remains a simple method, usually requiring a minimum of two procedures (including areola-nipple reconstruction) to create, in the majority of cases, a breast of acceptable symmetry and firmness. Patients who will not accept much scarring or who refuse major or multiple operations have been moderately satisfied with this method. It should be stressed that implantation requires more corrections of the opposite breast than other methods of reconstruction, and rarely creates large and ptotic breasts. This is least satisfactory in obese patients.

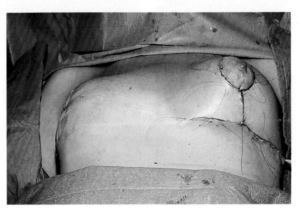

FIG. 2.6

Clinical Cases

Figures 2.7–2.17 show two implants placed simultaneously on both sides of a patient who had undergone bilateral mastectomies. At first the implants produced the same volume and shape; then capsular contracture became more pronounced on the left side, spoiling symmetry in volume, shape, and level. The surgeon has little influence on this phenomenon. After surgical capsulotomy, a second capsular contracture is likely to occur, but it is usually softer than the first *(Figs. 2.18– 2.22).*

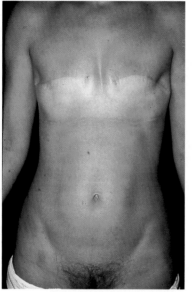

FIG. 2.7

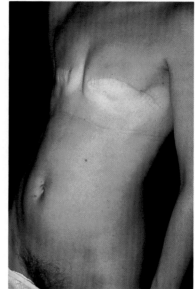

FIG. 2.8

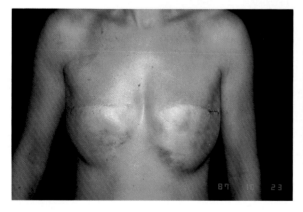

FIG. 2.9

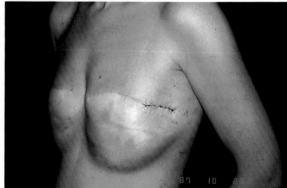

FIG. 2.10

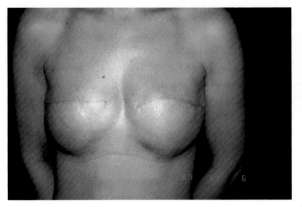

FIG. 2.11

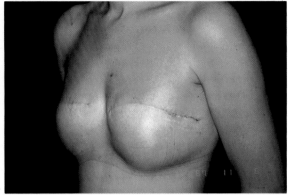

FIG. 2.12

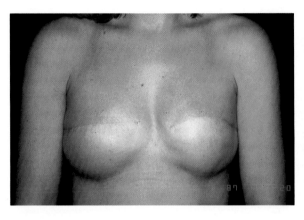

FIG. 2.13

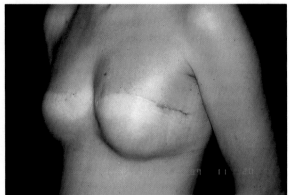

FIG. 2.14

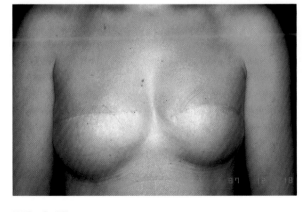

FIG. 2.15

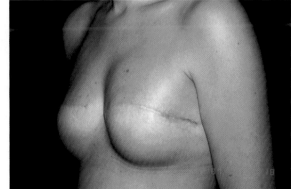

FIG. 2.16

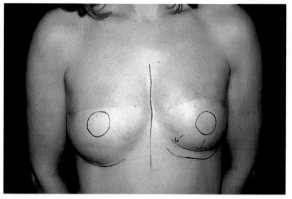

FIG. 2.17

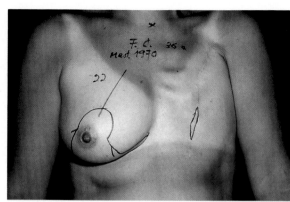

FIG. 2.18

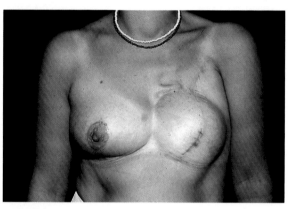

FIG. 2.19

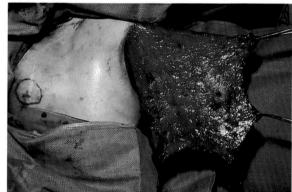

FIG. 2.20

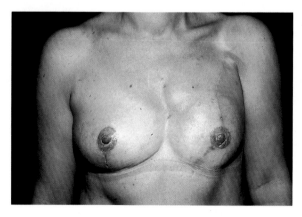

FIG. 2.21

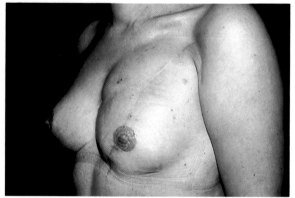

FIG. 2.22

The surgical results in the patient shown in *Figures 2.23 to 2.25* have not changed in 1 year after surgery. Of course, if the patient's weight changes, asymmetry of the breasts will follow. Sagging of the opposite breast may also partially spoil the result after some time. Every technique that involves implants, including expansion or latissimus reconstruction, has the same drawbacks. Only reconstructions with autogenous tissues are devoid of these problems.

BILATERAL RECONSTRUCTION OF THE BREAST WITH INSERTION OF SILICONE IMPLANTS

The objective in bilateral breast reconstruction is to obtain symmetry through the appropriate and equal placement of the inframammary fold and the creation of similar projections in both reconstructed breasts. This objective is not always easy to achieve, because bilateral mastectomies are seldom equal, especially in the amount of skin removed and the location of scars.

With the use of bilateral silicone implants, the reconstructed breasts tend to be round, thereby providing an equal measure of projection on both sides. Rarely is one able to obtain a semblance of ptosis, and the amount of capsular contracture is high but usually equal on both breasts.

In reconstructing the breasts by simple insertion of implants, the three key points comprise the creation of inframammary folds by advancement of the upper abdominal skin, partial coverage of the implants by the pectoralis major muscles, and increase in the transverse dimension of the chest skin to obtain more projection. These points are explained in detail in the following page.

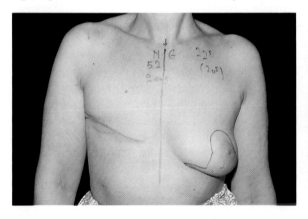

FIG. 2.23

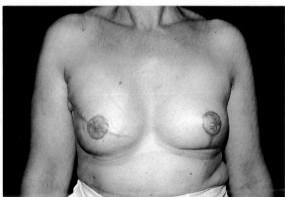

FIG. 2.24

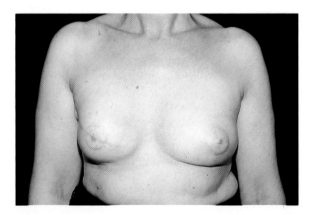

FIG. 2.25

Creation of the Inframammary Fold

In every method of breast reconstruction, particularly with the simple insertion of an implant, it is imperative to surgically create an inframammary fold. In a unilateral reconstruction, this fold should eventually be located at the same level as that on the contralateral normal side. In bilateral reconstruction, the folds should be at the same level. It is preferable to err on the side of placing the inframammary fold too low, because it can be raised by postoperative dressings or by the capsular contracture that is likely to occur. If the inframammary fold is too high, it will have to be lowered in a second operative procedure by dividing the capsule.

To correct the vertical skin deficit, we have found it helpful to undermine the upper abdominal skin and to advance it superiorly while fixing the inframammary fold with percutaneous sutures.

Muscle Coverage of the Implant

Although most writings on this subject suggest total muscle coverage of the implant, we have not found this to be essential. Obtaining coverage of the inferior half of the implant is difficult, and one is likely to place the implant too high in attempting to cover it with serratus muscle and/or the anterior rectus sheath.

Our method of reconstruction calls for placement of the implant under the pectoralis major muscle, thereby freeing the lower border of the muscle, as well as its fourth and fifth sternal origins. The free edge of the pectoralis major muscle is anchored to the subcutaneous tissue of the advanced upper abdominal skin. The implant's upper half is covered with muscle, but its lower portion is left uncovered and lies within a subcutaneous plane. Generally, the mastectomy scar lies over muscle and, consequently, is protected. In this way, one can place the implant at the proper level and, as the inframammary fold is fixed and more skin has been advanced superiorly to correct the vertical deficit, a certain amount of ptosis may occur as the implant and gravity stretch the overlying skin.

Obtaining Projection

The horizontal diameter of the chest wall—that is, the distance from the midsternum to the midaxillary line—determines the projection of the breast. If the patient has had a transverse incision, this distance can be increased by performing Z-plasties at the level of the scar. This not only will facilitate and break the visible transverse ridge, which the scar occasionally places over the implant, but it will also lengthen the horizontal line at the expense of the advanced upper abdominal skin. Two or three Z-plasties are sufficient and are usually done only on the skin, although occasionally the muscle must be freed in cases when the incision has extended through it. One should be careful not to place Z-plasties near the sternum for fear of hypertrophic scarring or because they may show in a low-cut dress or bathing suit.

Clinical Case

The following case demonstrates immediate reconstruction of the right breast and delayed reconstruction of the left postmastectomy side. The patient, a 27-year-old woman, had a left modified mastectomy for invasive intraductal carcinoma. On the right side, she had a biopsy-proven intraductal carcinoma *in situ*. A simple mastectomy was advised, as well as axillary sampling. On the left side, the modified mastectomy and axillary dissection were uneventful. On the right side, the mastectomy was performed by removing slightly less skin, and the axillary dissection was only a sampling procedure.

Our plan was to reconstruct both breasts immediately following the right mastectomy. It was done by advancing the upper abdominal skin, creating new inframammary folds, and performing Z-plasties along the transverse scar to increase the horizontal length of the scar.

The patient is seen preoperatively with the transverse mastectomy scar *(Figs. 2.26–2.28)*. The scar is relatively high in relation to the chest; it is raised, hypertrophic, and quite tight on this young, thin patient. The pectoralis major muscle is intact, without any atrophy, although she does have a slight concavity at the upper portion of the chest. The right breast is small, but normal, and an attempt will be made to do the mastectomy with an

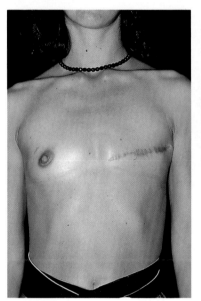

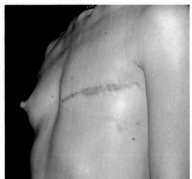

FIG. 2.27

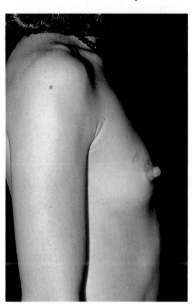

FIG. 2.26

FIG. 2.28

incision similar to the one on the left. The vertical and horizontal deficits are approximately 5 cm *(Figs. 2.29–2.31)*.

Following the right mastectomy and axillary sampling, bilateral reconstruction is performed. Location of the inframammary fold, the planning for the Z-plasties, and the determination of the projection should be done carefully, always striving for symmetry.

Surgical Technique

Reconstruction on the Left Side

The transverse mastectomy incision is opened laterally by delineating and incising a large Z-plasty. The incision is extended medially to facilitate undermining the upper abdominal skin. On this side, the pectoralis major muscle is attached to the skin. After performing the Z-plasty at the subcutaneous

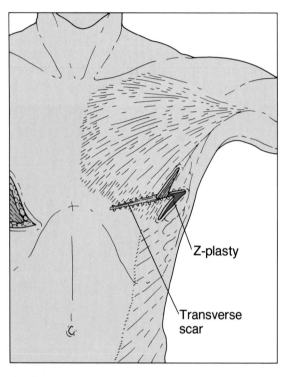
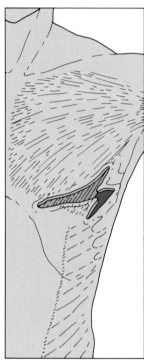
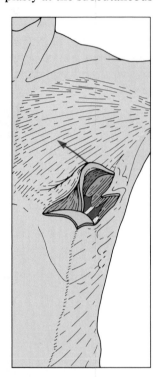

Z-plasty

Transverse scar

FIG. 2.29

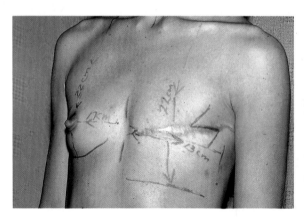

FIG. 2.30

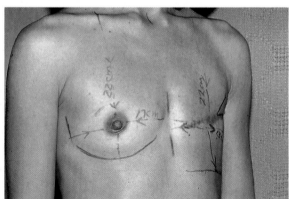

FIG. 2.31

tissue level and preserving the muscle intact, the lateral edge of the muscle is retracted and a pocket is created superiorly, medially, and inferiorly *(Fig. 2.29)*. The pocket should not be extended too far superiorly, for the implant will have a tendency to ride high. Inferiorly, however, the dissection should continue as far down as possible, over the serratus muscle and on top of the anterior rectus sheat *(Fig. 2.32)*. Hemostasis should be obtained carefully, for one can easily disrupt the perforating vessels from the epigastric arcade.

After the undermining, a breast implant sizer is used to determine the appropriate size for the patient's chest wall and amount of available skin. Temporary closure of the wound is performed with staples to check for adequate undermining superiorly, laterally, and inferiorly. One should be careful of excessive medial undermining in order to preserve most of the perforators from the internal mammary artery.

Once the appropriate implant size has been determined, the inframammary fold is fixed with percutaneous sutures of large nylon that attempt to approximate the skin and subcutaneous tissue to the underlying intercostal musculature *(Fig. 2.33)*. Care should be exercised to make sure that one does not introduce the needle intrathoracically. In delineating this inframammary fold, one should create a curve with its convexity pointing downwards and with its medial and lateral edges higher than the central point. Trial and error is necessary for this procedure, and we have not found any absolute ways to facilitate it. In some cases, one may place the percutaneous sutures with the implant sizer in place, but most of the time it must be removed after determining the approximate level where the inframammmary fold should be placed. Other methods have been tried, such as tattooing with methylene blue or counting the ribs and intercostal spaces. Although these steps are helpful, they are not infallible.

Once the inframammary fold has been marked with percutaneous sutures, the fold should be anchored by placing deep sutures with 3.0 nylon, connecting the subcutaneous tissue of the upper abdominal flap to the chest wall. Again, the percutaneous sutures serve as guides. We have always found it helpful to place the deep sutures even

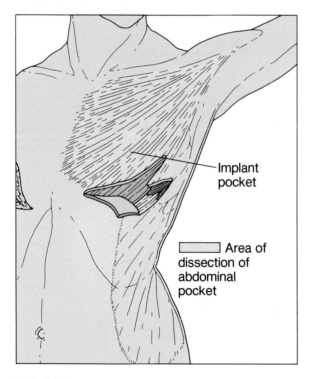

FIG. 2.32

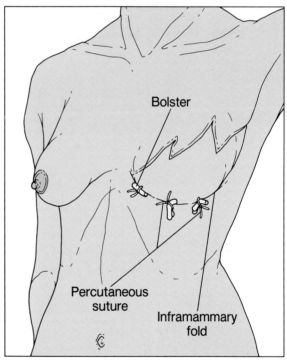

FIG. 2.33

lower than the percutaneous ones to further advance the upper abdominal skin and to place the inframammary fold low. Chapter 9 shows the percutaneous creation of an inframammary fold which may also be applicable to this method of reconstruction.

A temporary sizer implant is placed and the wound temporarily closed with staples as we turn our attention to reconstruction of the other side.

Reconstruction on the Right Side

On this side we have an acceptable mastectomy defect with undisturbed underlying pectoralis musculature. Superiorly, the skin undermining extends almost to the clavicle, and laterally to the anterior border of the latissimus dorsi muscle. Inferiorly, a portion of the anterior rectus sheath is exposed.

Two aspects of this procedure are different from

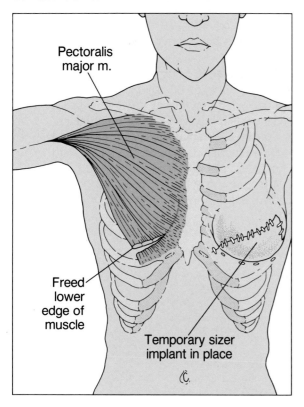

FIG. 2.34

Pectoralis major m.

Freed lower edge of muscle

Temporary sizer implant in place

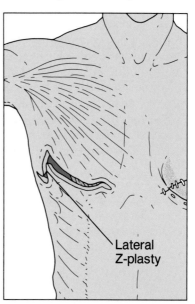

Lateral Z-plasty

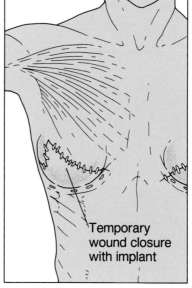

Temporary wound closure with implant

FIG. 2.35

the reconstruction on the other side. First, we attempt to close the wound laterally and superiorly to prevent migration of the implant either laterally to the axilla or too far superiorly. Second, we free the lower edge of the pectoralis major muscle and suture it under normal tension to the subcutaneous tissue of the advanced upper abdominal skin.

The upper abdominal flap is dissected inferiorly on top of the anterior rectus sheath to approximately the same level as the contralateral one. The lower edge of the pectoralis muscle is freed and its lowermost origins from the sternum are divided, thus providing a free inferior border of the muscle *(Fig. 2.34)*. The silicone implant sizer, the same size as the contralateral one, is inserted. With the sizer in place, one determines the level at which the superior and axillary pockets should be closed with 3.0 nylon.

A Z-plasty, which will increase the horizontal length of the scar, is performed laterally in the transverse mastectomy scar. With the implant sizer in place, temporary closure of the wound is performed with staples *(Fig. 2.35)*. The percutaneous sutures are placed to equal the inframammary fold on the contralateral side. This is the most difficult and critical portion of the procedure. Once the sutures are placed with the patient in a supine position, the anesthesiologist should sit her up as much as possible to determine symmetry as to projection and level. Although the same implant size is satisfactory in most cases, one should not hesitate to use different size implants to obtain equal projection.

If we are satisfied with the delineation of the inframammary folds by percutaneous and deep sutures of 3.0 nylon, we suture the lower edge of the pectoralis muscle to the subcutaneous tissue of the advanced upper abdominal skin *(Fig. 2.36)*.

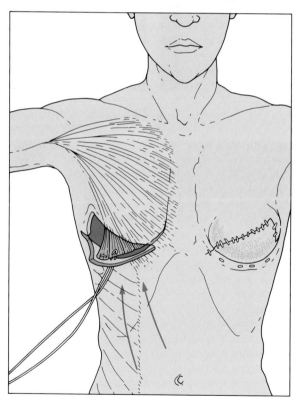

FIG. 2.36

The permanent implants are inserted. We have found the low profile implant to be helpful for these cases. Double lumen or polyurethane-covered implants may also be used.

Suction catheters are placed on both sides. Two catheters may be needed on the immediately reconstructed side because a potential for the accumulation of fluid along the axilla exists. The wounds are closed and a bulky type of figure 8 circumferential dressing is applied.

The patient, shown postoperatively and prior to nipple reconstruction *(Figs. 2.37–2.39),* has satis-

factory projection. Despite our efforts, some disparity in the inframammary fold level is present; the right side is higher than the left, due to the greater degree of capsular contracture. This biologic and, in most cases, unpredictable factor, is the reason for our emphasis in placing the inframammary fold low. The Z-plasty on the right side, placed laterally, can be covered by clothing.

The patient is shown after the bilateral nipple reconstruction *(Figs. 2.40–2.43).* The scars remain red. A decision was made not to lower the inframammary fold on the right side because, in our

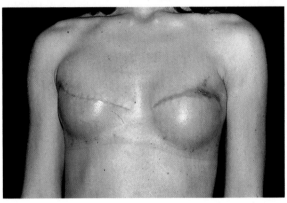

FIG. 2.37

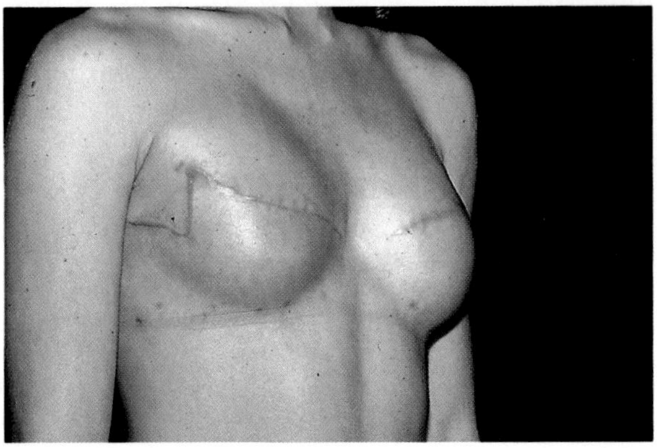

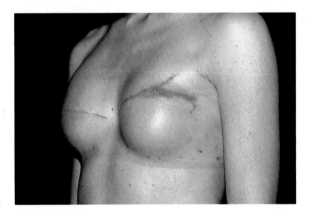

FIG. 2.38

FIG. 2.39

experience, efforts to correct relatively small defects are likely to fail, sometimes making the defect worse.

RECONSTRUCTION WITH SKIN EXPANDERS

Inflatable Tissue Expander

Reconstruction using an inflatable tissue expander (ITE) is indicated after a modified radical mastectomy in which limited skin and muscle cover do

not permit an adequate cosmetic result with the use of a silicone gel implant. An undeniable advantage of the expander technique is the planned two-stage reconstruction.

Surgical Technique

Delayed Reconstruction

The mastectomy scar is opened approximately 4 to 6 cm. This incision is usually situated over the pectoralis major muscle. By using blunt dissection, a submuscular pocket is formed that extends lat-

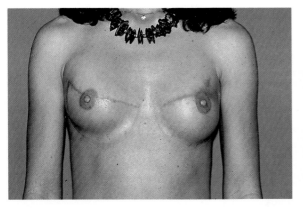

FIG. 2.40

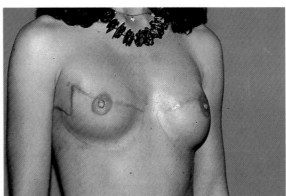

FIG. 2.41

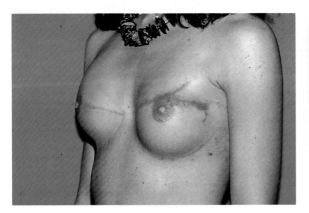

FIG. 2.42

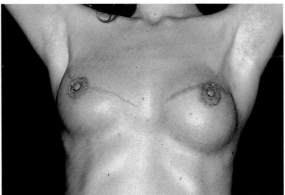

FIG. 2.43

erally to the midaxillary line, superiorly to a level just higher than the opposite breast, and medially to the border of the sternum *(Fig. 2.44)*. Inferiorly, the dissection is subcutaneous and extends over the costal margin. It is imperative that the expander be placed low, for the capsular contracture will bring it up. An early mistake in our experience was to place the expander too high.

Immediate Reconstruction

The ITE is inserted in one of two ways: the serratus anterior method, or the pectoralis major and subcutaneous lower dissection.

SERRATUS ANTERIOR METHOD. The dissection of the pocket commences through a vertical incision into the serratus anterior, 4 cm lateral

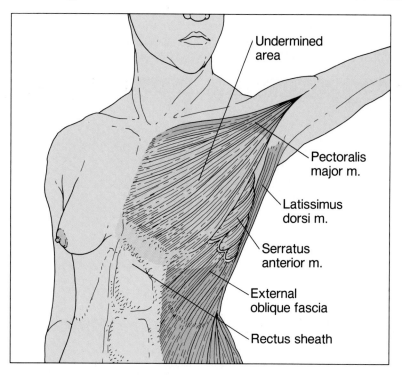

Undermined area

Pectoralis major m.

Latissimus dorsi m.

Serratus anterior m.

External oblique fascia

Rectus sheath

FIG. 2.44

to the pectoralis major. Sharp dissection is required where the fibers of the pectoralis major and serratus muscles are attached to the ribs and lead to the plane under the pectoralis. This method, although bloodier, has the advantage of providing total muscle cover for the expander. One should always be conscious of placing the expander low enough.

PECTORALIS MAJOR AND SUBCUTANEOUS LOWER DISSECTION.   As with the delayed reconstruction technique, the pectoralis major can be retracted or occasionally split in the line of its

fibers and the submuscular pocket created, as described previously *(Fig. 2.45)*. In each method the injection dome is brought to lie in a subcutaneous position where it can easily be palpable and accessible for percutaneous injection, as well as subsequent easy removal.

On a separate table free from sharp objects or needles, the expander implant should be filled with 50 cc of saline and checked for leaks. Subsequently, after dissecting a large, low pocket, the expander implant is inserted and, after properly shortening, the tubing is connected with the injec-

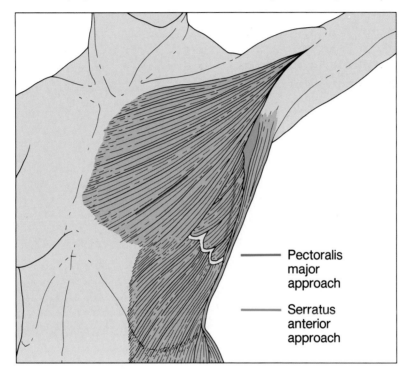

Pectoralis major approach

Serratus anterior approach

FIG. 2.45

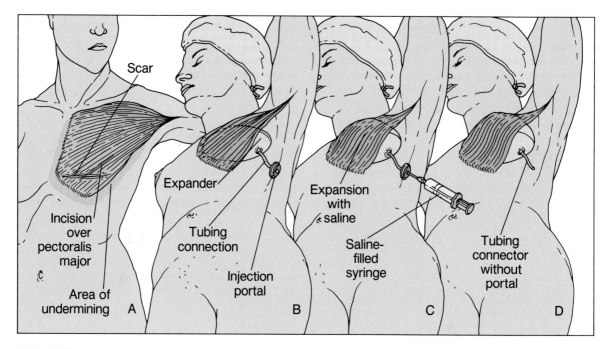

Scar

Incision over pectoralis major

Area of undermining

A

Expander

Tubing connection

Injection portal

B

Expansion with saline

Saline-filled syringe

C

Tubing connector without portal

D

FIG. 2.46

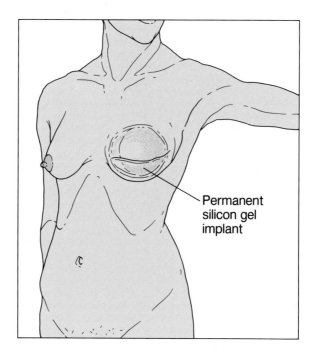

Permanent silicon gel implant

FIG. 2.47

tion portal. It is necessary to tie the tubing securely to the groove in the adaptor with a 2.0 silk suture *(Fig. 2.46.A–D)*.

A separate pocket is dissected subcutaneously to house the injection portal away from the expander. It should be placed so as to avoid inadvertent puncture of the expander. Suggested locations for the injection portal are the midaxillary line, the lateral costal margin, or, rarely, the midsternum.

After closure of all the wounds, we advise that the expander be inflated percutaneously through the injection portal with an additional 100 to 150 cc of saline. This maneuver flattens the expander and avoids wrinkles or folds, assures that the portal is not upside down, and creates a small breast mound.

Postoperative Care

One or 2 weeks are allowed for healing of the wound before further inflation of the ITE. We use an average of 50-ml aliquots of saline injected with 23- or 25-gauge needles. This is repeated every week until the expander appears larger than the opposite breast. This usually takes 6 to 8 weeks. To facilitate inflation in the office, a 250-cc saline bag is hung on an IV pole and the solution injected into the portal.

At the time of injection, the capillary return of the skin is carefully checked before continuing with further inflation. Pain is usually the limiting factor as to the inflatable volume in each session.

When there is doubt about the viability of the expanded skin, fluid is withdrawn from the injection dome. Whenever possible, we wait at least 3 to 6 months from the time at which the desired inflated size is achieved before proceeding with surgical insertion of a permanent prosthesis *(Fig. 2.47)*. This prevents the "recall" phenomenon that usually produces shrinkage of the expanded skin. The ITE is inflated to a volume ranging from 250 to 1,000 cubic centimeters.

Complications

The complications associated with the ITE are described in Table 2.1.

THE LOWER THORACIC ADVANCEMENT FLAP IN BREAST RECONSTRUCTION (RYAN-PENNISI METHOD)

The Ryan-Pennisi method of reconstruction addresses two important principles that help in obtaining symmetry with the contralateral breast. First, it adds skin in the vertical dimension by advancing the upper abdominal skin (usually in excess). Second, it creates a fixed inframammary fold, which permits the overlying skin to stretch and to develop a semblance of ptosis thereby simulating a more normal breast.

The disadvantages relate to the difficulty of determining the exact level of the inframammary

Table 2.1
Inflatable Tissue Expander (ITE) Complications

MECHANICAL	Disruption, injection dome leak, inversion of the injection portal, expander leaks or rupture
TECHNICAL	Skin necrosis, extrusion of inflatable tissue expander
SELF-INFLICTED	Deflation from pin pricks
CHEST WALL	Deformities are not common following tissue expansion, but may be caused by multiple rib fractures of the anterior thorax, especially in the osteoporotic postmenopausal female

line intraoperatively, and of creating a tight and tenuous suture line (the inframammary line) that may result in exposure of the silicone implant.

This procedure is illustrated on a young patient who had a modified mastectomy with preservation of the pectoralis major muscle, adequate skin in the upper abdomen, and a contralateral breast that was somewhat enlarged and pendulous, requiring reduction.

Figure 2.48.A,B shows the lateral and anterior

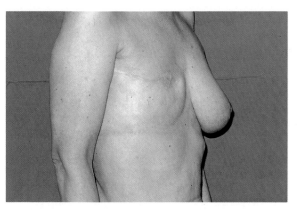

FIG. 2.48.A

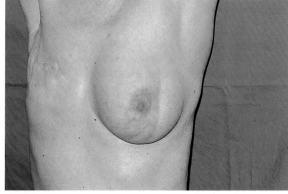

FIG. 2.48.B

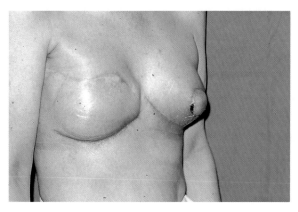

FIG. 2.49.A

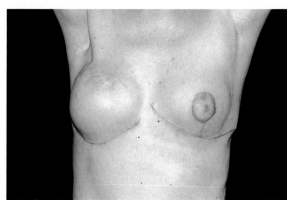

FIG. 2.49.B

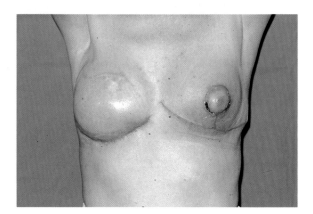

FIG. 2.49.C

BREAST RECONSTRUCTION WITH IMPLANTS AND EXPANDERS

views of the patient before surgery. The vertical dimple line on the left breast is the end result of Mondor's disease. A considerable amount of upper abdominal skin was available that could be advanced superiorly to create the inframammary fold. *Figures 2.49.A–C* and *2.50.A, B* show the end result following the Ryan-Pennisi advancement procedure. The newly created inframammary fold is at the same level as the contralateral one. A small reduction and mastopexy were performed on the opposite breast for symmetry.

The steps of the procedure are illustrated in *Figure 2.51*. The patient, in the lateral position, demonstrates the transverse mastectomy scar which is considerably higher than the contralateral inframammary fold. The center drawing reveals the location of the inframammary fold, and the drawing on the right shows the creation of the inframam-

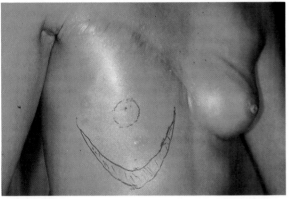

FIG. 2.50.A *(Figure 2.50.A,B courtesy of Dr. Vincent Pennisi, St. Francis Hospital, San Francisco, California.)*

FIG. 2.50.B

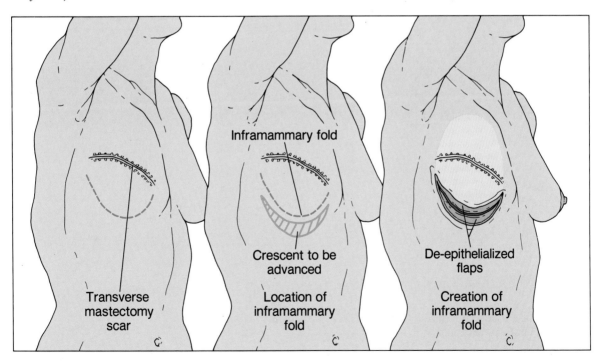

Inframammary fold

Crescent to be advanced

De-epithelialized flaps

Transverse mastectomy scar

Location of inframammary fold

Creation of inframammary fold

FIG. 2.51

mary fold at the proper level by advancement of the upper abdominal skin and de-epithelialization of 1 to 2 cm of the upper and lower flaps.

Figure 2.52 shows the lower flap portion which has been de-epithelialized and sutured to the sixth intercostal space while the upper flap is dissected to create an adequate pocket for insertion of the implant. The inset in the left drawing shows the de-epithelialized portion of the lower flap being sutured either to the intercostal space or to the periosteum of the rib, preferably the former. The upper flap, a portion of which is also de-epithelialized, is to be sutured over the lower flap. The drawing on the right shows the completed procedure—with the inset of the upper and lower flaps creating the submammary fold and with sutures approximated to support the implant.

Surgical Technique

Planning begins with the patient seated and preferably wearing a brassiere to demonstrate the level of the inframammary line on the normal as well as on the mastectomy side. One advances the upper abdominal skin and gets an idea of its looseness.

After marking the inframammary fold which corresponds to the line of the brassiere, a crescent is marked approximately 2 cm wide in its central portion, usually at the midclavicular line (*Fig. 2.51, center*). It extends from a medial point at which the opposite inframammary fold would terminate and runs laterally to the anterior axillary line. The location of the crescent *below* the inframammary fold is variable from 2 to 6 cm depending on the looseness of the upper abdominal skin. The more one can advance, the more skin will be available in the upper chest to admit a larger prosthesis which will stretch the skin and result in more ptosis. The lower one places the crescent from the inframammary line, however, the more one is creating dog ears at the medial and lateral points which need to be corrected at the completion of the procedure.

The location of the inframammary fold is difficult to determine intraoperatively. We have made attempts to tattoo it percutaneously with needles and methylene blue or to count the ribs and intercostal spaces, comparing it with the opposite breast. All have been only partly successful. The anterior thoracic skin ascends when the patient re-

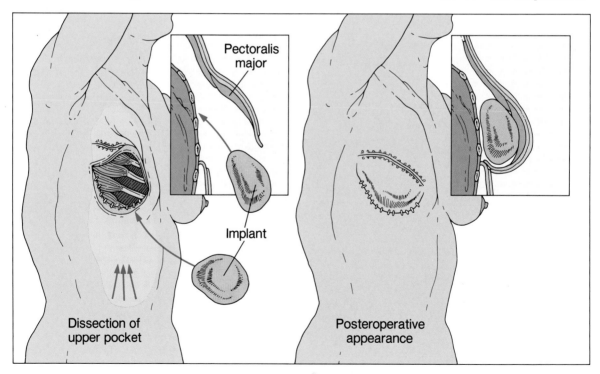

FIG. 2.52

clines, and it is even higher when the arm and shoulder are abducted. In every case, it is advisable in the middle of the procedure to sit the patient up to check not only on the size of the breast mound but also on the location of the inframammary fold.

Once the markings have been made with the patient in the semisitting position, the marked crescent is de-epithelialized and a full thickness incision is made, bisecting it in its entire length. The upper chest flap is then elevated underneath the pectoralis major muscle, but on top of the serratus anterior muscle. The lower chest flap is also elevated at the deep subcutaneous level over the anterior rectus sheath. The lower dissection extends toward the costal margin for a distance of 6 to 15 cm depending on the degree of advancement. The inferior flap is then advanced in the superomedial direction and sutured to the chest wall with permanent nylon sutures. To avoid sutures in the periosteum that at times can be painful to the patient, we prefer to suture the flap to the intercostal space.

A silicone sizer implant is placed and a temporary closure is made approximating the upper flap to the lower one. The patient is then raised to a sitting position for a check of the size of the breast mound and the location of the inframammary fold.

It is preferable to err on the side of making the fold slightly lower rather than too high. Rarely, a lowered inframammary fold may be chosen purposely if the opposite breast is quite ptotic and the patient does not allow it to be adjusted.

Once the proper silicone implant is placed, the upper chest flap is sutured to the de-epithelialized portion of the lower flap with fine nylon in as broad a dermal apposition as possible. This step constitutes the weakest portion of the suture line, which at times results in exposure of the implant. Dog-ears, by necessity, will appear on the medial and the lateral aspect of the incision, and they must be minimized either by excising portions of the skin or by de-epithelializing and burying them medially where they will create an abnormal bulge. An elastic-type figure 8 dressing is applied. It is replaced in a few days by a brassiere.

If an alteration is necessary on the opposite breast, it can be done at the same time or at a second sitting when the nipple is reconstructed. There are advantages and disadvantages with either choice. We prefer to reduce or do a ptosis procedure at the same time as the reconstruction, so that any final adjustment can be easily done at the time of nipple reconstruction.

When performing a reduction or a ptosis procedure on the contralateral breast, one should keep in mind that (in reducing or raising a breast) the inframammary fold appears raised on the operating table. At the end of the procedure, one is likely to produce a lower inframammary fold on the reconstructed breast than on the breast that has been reduced or ptosed. In time, the inframammary line on the reduced breast will fall to the previous level, while on the reconstructed breast it is likely to rise due to capsular contracture. In these cases, if one achieves symmetric inframammary lines at the time of surgery, the end result will be unsatisfactory.

The Ryan-Pennisi procedure has given excellent results and has the added advantage of stretching the overlying skin over the fixed inframammary fold slowly, resulting in improvement over a period of 6 months to a year with some ptosis as well as a teardrop appearance of the reconstructed breast.

We have discontinued performing this procedure, but use its principle in our reconstructions. The modification we use avoids the inframammary incision. We advance the upper abdominal skin and fix it to the chest wall and intercostal space with deeply buried sutures, approaching the reconstruction through the same mastectomy scar.

Modification of the Ryan-Pennisi Procedure

In the modified procedure, the same mastectomy scar is used and reopened. The upper chest flap is also elevated underneath the pectoralis major muscle while the lower one is undermined toward the costal margin at the deep subcutaneous plane. As the surgeon applies traction to the upper abdominal flap, a line is drawn to simulate the inframammary line, approximately 2 to 3 cm below the contralateral one. As traction is maintained superiorly, temporary percutaneous sutures of 0 nylon are placed through the skin and into the intercostal space, fixing it in a gentle curve from the parasternal line to the anterior axillary line. A total of three or four of the sutures are placed but left untied. These serve as guides and will indicate the level at which the deep subcutaneous tissue is to be anchored to the intercostal space.

With the upper abdominal flap tractioned superiorly, the surgeon then approximates the subcutaneous tissue of the upper abdominal flap to the intercostal space in the same gentle curve and slightly below the percutaneous sutures. As much upper abdominal skin as possible is brought up, and a new inframammary fold is created. Horizontal mattress sutures of 3.0 nylon are used, and care is taken to avoid puckering the overlying skin. We prefer this approach (the percutaneous sutures serving as guidelines) to other methods of tattooing with needles because it seems to be easier and more reliable.

The appropriately sized implant is then inserted. If the mastectomy scar is quite thick and deep, one may perform a lateral Z-plasty to increase the transverse diameter at the time of the closure. The Z-plasty should not be done if there is any question about the viability of the skin flaps or if it would put the implant in jeopardy by exposing it. This modification has the advantage of avoiding the extra scar in the inframammary fold as well as the medial and lateral dog-ears, but the exact location of the inframammary fold is just as difficult

in the modification as in the Ryan-Pennisi procedure. Efforts are concentrated on making the inframammary fold 1 to 2 cm lower than the contralateral one.

The percutaneous placement of the temporary sutures should be done carefully to avoid intrathoracic puncture (which has not occurred but could theoretically occur). The percutaneous sutures are either removed or they can be tied over a gauze bolster to be removed in 3 to 5 days to avoid any cross-hatching on the skin.

BILATERAL RECONSTRUCTION WITH SIMPLE PLACEMENT OF IMPLANTS IN AN OBESE PATIENT

As a general rule, unilateral reconstruction with the placement of silicone implants in an obese patient yields unsatisfactory results because of the inability to match the opposite breast, despite procedures such as reduction mammaplasty on the remaining breast. There seems to be an impossibility in the majority of obese patients to form a

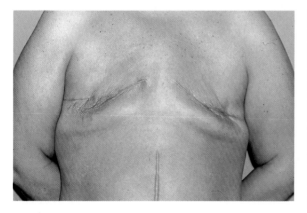

FIG. 2.53

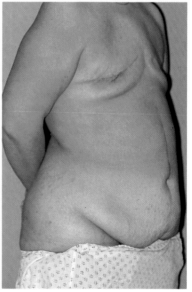

FIG. 2.54

well-defined breast mound with satisfactory projection. Even if it forms, the breast mound is round and does not have the ptotic appearance of the normal breast.

In the bilateral reconstructions, however, symmetry can be obtained through the placement of identical breast implants, particularly if the mastectomy incisions are similar.

Clinical Case

A 55-year-old moderately obese woman had mastectomies approximately 20 years ago for an undetermined pathology not proven to be carcinoma. She wanted a relatively straightforward reconstruction and, at the same time, she wished to get rid of her abdominal panniculus. She would have been a good candidate for the bilateral transverse island abdominal flap, but this procedure was not chosen.

Examination of the preoperative stage *(Figs. 2.53, 2.54)* shows the effects of the mastectomy through transverse incisions. Note the persistence of the symmetric inframammary folds as well as the axillary fullness. She does have a large abdom-

inal panniculus with a long midline scar from previous gastrointestinal surgery.

The procedure consisted of the symmetric insertion of 450-cc silicone gel implants bilaterally by opening the previous mastectomy scars. In an effort to obtain further projection, two Z-plasties were performed to lengthen the transverse scar. An effort was made not to dissect the pocket any lower or to disturb the inframammary folds. During the original procedure, an abdominoplasty was performed. By using a transverse incision, we took advantage of the midline incision to decrease the transverse girth and thus delineate the waist better.

Figures 2.55, 2.56 show the patient months later after the bilateral areola and nipple reconstruction.

A corollary from this case would indicate that, whenever possible, it is better to reconstruct both breasts with a similar method and procedure. If one is performing a mastectomy on the opposite breast, it is suggested that it be done through a similar incision and, preferably, that it be a simple mastectomy rather than a subcutaneous one. When two different mastectomies have been performed, the problems of symmetry are compounded.

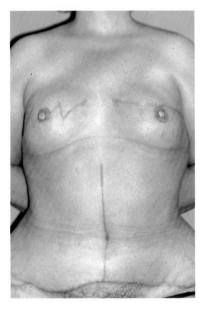

FIG. 2.55

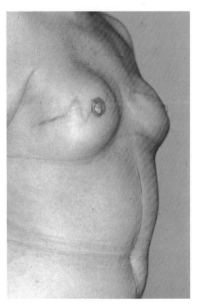

FIG. 2.56

CHAPTER·3

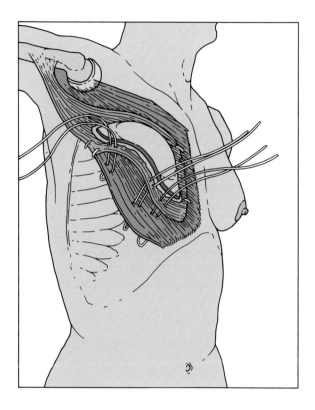

Breast Reconstruction with Latissimus Dorsi Myocutaneous Flap

The latissimus dorsi myocutaneous flap is a reliable breast reconstruction method that can be performed in a single stage. Relatively easy and safe to execute, this method is versatile enough to accomplish the requirements of most breast reconstructions. The disadvantage is that it leaves a scar on the back which is less acceptable to patients than the lower transverse abdominal scar. This method, however, provides an island of skin as well as muscle which can be transposed from the back to the front of the chest, as a pendulum pivoting at the thoracodorsal vessels and at the insertion of the latissimus dorsi muscle in the humerus. In most cases, a silicone implant needs to be inserted at the same time to simulate the breast mound.

The principles and guidelines of breast reconstruction with the latissimus dorsi muscle will be discussed from the viewpoints of the donor site, the recipient site, the shape and orientation of the skin island, and the placement of the skin island in the front of the chest.

Principles

The latissimus muscle is a fan-shaped muscle extending over the back from the lower six thoracic spines and the iliac crest to the proximal third of the humerus. It is an adductor of the arm. Its major blood supply and innervation are from the axilla. Rotation of the muscle around the thoracic wall to the breast region is thus possible without jeopardizing its neurovascular supply.

After dividing the peripheral origin of the muscle and preserving the thoracodorsal artery and the nerve, this unit, which includes an ellipse of overlying skin, is carefully rotated on its humeral insertion toward the breast region under a bridge of thoracic skin below the axilla. This provides additional skin to replace that removed during the mastectomy, and additional muscle to simulate the pectoralis major.

The quantity of skin taken with the muscle is often insufficient to replace the skin of the missing breast, and the latissimus dorsi muscle is much thinner than the pectoralis. One should take as much skin as is compatible with direct closure of the donor wound. The skin ellipse may be placed anywhere on the muscle, but it should be understood that, after transposition, the skin island orientation changes. For example, a transversely oriented skin island becomes vertical in the chest. Or, if the skin is taken on the lower part of the muscle, it will be placed higher after rotation. The skin island placement depends on the type of mastectomy. A cloth or paper pattern, which is allowed to pivot at the axilla, is useful for visualizing this change.

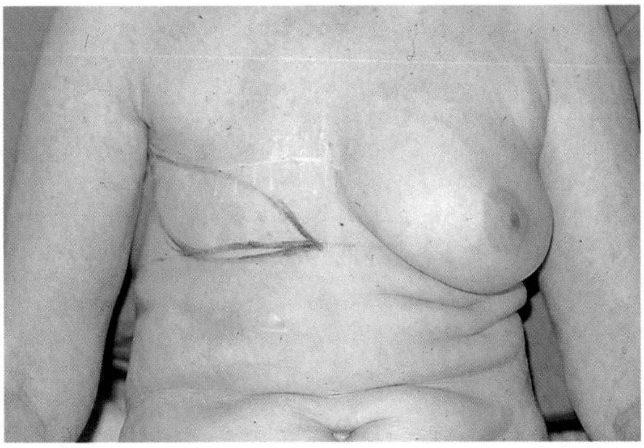

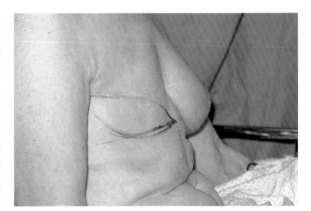

FIG. 3.1

FIG. 3.2

The whole latissimus dorsi muscle is not always necessary for the reconstruction. Part of it can be left in place, but this remaining part will atrophy. Taking the total muscle requires a large dorsal undermining, causes more bleeding, and increases the risk of seroma formation. Consequently, the muscle is taken totally or almost totally only if the pectoralis muscle has been removed or denervated. If the pectoralis muscle is intact, more of the latissimus dorsi muscle is left behind. Muscle should be retained beyond the border of the skin

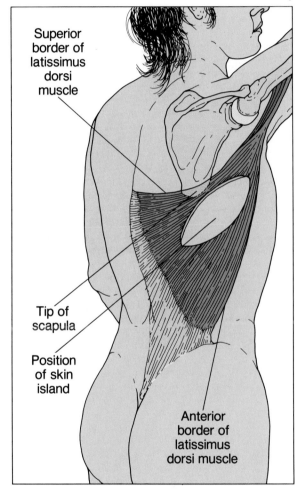

Superior
border of
latissimus
dorsi
muscle

Tip of
scapula

Position
of skin
island

Anterior
border of
latissimus
dorsi muscle

FIG. 3.3

island, even when it is outlined transversely just below the tip of the scapula.

Planning is essential and should start on the evening before the operation. With the patient standing, the pattern should be written out. The best aesthetic placement for the skin island is transverse and below the scapula.

To place the dorsal skin flap in the correct position, the upper limit of the patient's brassiere is located, and the upper border of the skin island is drawn a little lower as a smooth curve. The flap extends for 15 to 20 cm, but does not reach the midline where the trapezius muscle covers the origin of the latissimus. The lower border of the skin island is more angular and convex caudally, to create more projection of the breast after rotation. The width of the flap is determined (it usually measures 6 to 8 cm). The flap should be as wide as possible, but without impairing direct suturing of the donor site. One should remember that the skin is under tension, and a 6-cm skin island becomes a 10-cm defect.

The skin island ellipse is transposed to the chest and invariably is placed vertically or in a lazy S configuration, often disregarding the transverse mastectomy scar. The objective is to add to the transverse diameter by the vertical placement of the skin island. The lower end of the skin island should form part of the inframammary fold.

Surgical Technique

The inframammary fold is marked on the normal side and the pattern is transferred to the mastectomy side with the patient sitting *(Figs. 3.1, 3.2)*. At the same time the anterior border of the latissimus dorsi muscle, as well as the tip of the scapula on the mastectomy side, are drawn for guidance *(Fig. 3.3)*. The mastectomy scar is noted and the muscle is evaluated for paralysis. One may mistakenly think that the innervation of the latissimus dorsi muscle is intact by a hypertrophied teres major muscle, but, if the latissimus dorsi muscle is denervated, a slight winging of the scapula may be noted, even when the long thoracic nerve innervating the serratus anterior muscle is intact.

The patient is placed on the operating table in a semilateral position exposing the entire "hemiback" and the chest, including the opposite breast. The use of the "beanbag" to position the patient has been a great help to avoid abnormal pressure points. This positioning allows the entire reconstruction to be performed without changing the patient's position or redraping. Checking for symmetry with the patient sitting up, however, is not possible.

The skin island is outlined over the latissimus dorsi muscle in the proper shape and direction, as determined by the preplanned reconstructive objective. The incisions are made and the skin flaps elevated sharply while the assistant forcefully retracts the skin with skin hooks superiorly and inferiorly, as well as anteriorly and laterally. Gentle traction may be used on the skin island itself without fear of disrupting the perforating vessels. Anchoring stitches are not necessary between the muscle and overlying skin, because of the forceful attachment of the skin to the underlying muscle. Elevation of the skin flaps becomes bloody as one approaches the midline of the back because of the paravertebral perforators. Dissection may be difficult in the anterior border of the latissimus dorsi muscle because of scarring from the mastectomy.

After the skin flaps are elevated, the latissimus dorsi muscle and its overlying skin island are ready to be freed. Freeing the muscle starts away from previous areas of scarring. It is best begun at the superior border of the latissimus dorsi muscle by first identifying the tip of the scapula and realizing that the superior border of the muscle extends approximately 2 cm above it (Fig. 3.4). Allis clamps are used to elevate the edge of the muscle. By blunt and sharp dissection, its undersurface is found

without difficulty. Finger dissection continues, and the muscle and skin islands are elevated in a bloodless field.

As the dissection proceeds, the anterior border of the latissimus dorsi muscle is noted. The two borders can be easily connected, avoiding the inclusion of portions of the serratus anterior muscle. The muscle is then divided along its tendinous origin near the midline. This is a relatively bloody dissection because of the paravertebral vessels, which should be hemostatically controlled.

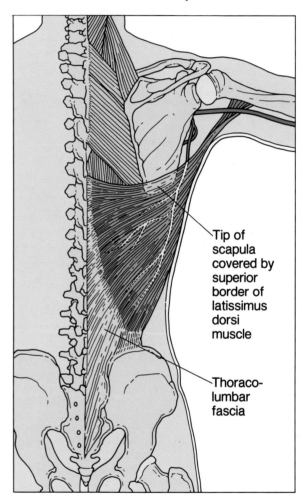

Tip of scapula covered by superior border of latissimus dorsi muscle

Thoraco-lumbar fascia

FIG. 3.4

As one retracts the inferior skin flap, a decision is made as to how much of the muscle should be included. A transverse cut is made from the anterior border of the latissimus dorsi muscle to join the vertical cut along the midline of the back, freeing the unit from its medial, posterior, and inferior attachments. The dissection continues superiorly toward the insertion of the muscle and its vascular pedicle. Along the posterior axillary line, one finds perforators which are divided between hemoclips. It is best to continue the dissection superiorly and posteriorly along the tip of the scapula, which is a safer place, rather than in the anterior axilla, until one identifies the thoracodorsal vessels. Once these are identified, the dissection continues toward the insertion of the muscle so that every attachment is freed, and the whole unit can be moved as a pendulum on a relatively narrow pivot point.

Several points should be kept in mind during the dissection.

1. The dissection is made *under* the latissimus dorsi muscle to avoid inadvertent elevation of the skin island from the muscle. This is ensured by starting the dissection superiorly just above the tip of the scapula.
2. The serratus anterior muscle is *not* included with the flap. However, it may inadvertently be included if the dissection starts at the anterior border of the latissimus dorsi muscle because of scarring. One should note the direction of the fibers of the serratus anterior muscle, which are almost perpendicular to those of the latissimus dorsi muscle.
3. The superior border of the latissimus dorsi muscle extends above the tip of the scapula and superficial to it. If one finds oneself underneath the scapula, the plane of dissection is too deep.
4. The latissimus dorsi muscle has a tendinous origin from the dorsal spine, and one must be careful not to cut too deeply and include the paravertebral muscle, the fibers of which are oriented cephalocaudally. Two rows of paravertebral perforators are found in this region, and should be ligated as they are divided.
5. The inferior transection of the muscle is facilitated by applying superior traction on the muscle. If there is concern about hemostasis, the transection should be done between clamps to avoid blood loss. Most of the bleeding occurs during elevation of the skin and muscle unit, and is most likely to occur posteriorly with the paravertebral perforators. Once all the borders of the muscle are divided, Allis clamps are placed on the anterior, posterior, and inferior borders. With the assistant holding up the myocutaneous unit, the perforating vessels from the chest wall are easily seen and divided between hemoclips.
6. Scarring from the mastectomy will be present on the anterior border of the latissimus dorsi muscle. Careful dissection is necessary, and a good knowledge of the anatomy of the thoracodorsal vessels is important. The latter sends a large branch to supply the serratus anterior muscle and will be the pivoting point of the unit. Rarely, this branch may need to be divided to make the flap pivot higher. The thoracodorsal vessel itself enters the muscle and almost immediately divides into two branches which diverge toward the anterior and posterior portions of the muscle.
7. The insertion of the latissimus dorsi muscle is left undisturbed on most occasions. If it needs to be divided, this may be accomplished by identifying and protecting the vascular pedicle, and then dissecting enough above it so that a finger may be used to encircle the tendinous insertion, which may then be divided.

Closure of the Back Wound

The flap is transposed anteriorly and the back wound is closed in layers with fine nylon. At least one or two suction catheters are placed and brought out through the ends of the incision. Separate stab wounds for the exiting of the suction catheters may be necessary.

Anterior Chest Wall Dissection

The marked inframammary line and mastectomy incision are noted. The decision is made to use the previous scar or to create a new one. Based on the

principles of projection and ptosis, it is helpful to place the myocutaneous unit over the chest wall to determine how and where the skin flap is going to lie comfortably and to provide the needed projection or ptosis. The unit usually lies best in an oblique position, with the vertical component along the anterior axilla line and the most medial extent reaching the inframammary fold and creating a J- or lazy S-type arrangement.

Because most patients with modified mastectomies have a transverse incision, this scar is disregarded. A J-type incision is made almost over the entire length of the skin island starting above the transverse scar and extending toward the infra-

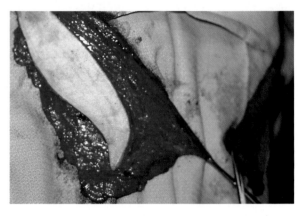

FIG. 3.6

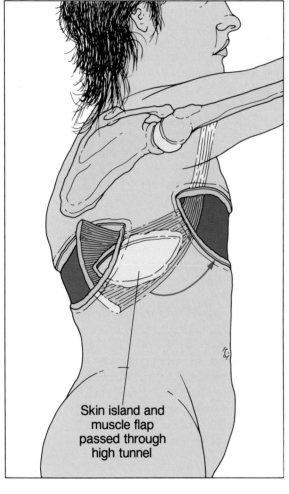

Skin island and muscle flap passed through high tunnel

FIG. 3.5

mammary fold, which is opened medially as far as the skin island will reach. Leaving a bridge of uncut skin superiorly will facilitate closure. The skin island is passed through a high tunnel, and one avoids connecting the posterior wound with the anterior wound in its entirety *(Figs. 3.5, 3.6)*. This is essential, for it will prevent migration of the implant posteriorly.

Once the chest incision is made, skin flaps are elevated superiorly, laterally, and inferiorly. The superior flap is elevated under the pectoralis major muscle. The lateral one is elevated to the midaxillary line. The inferior flap is elevated 2 or 3 cm below the marked inframammary line. Low placement is important because of the expected capsular contracture, but it should not be so low as to produce an unsightly bulge of the latissimus skin island inferiorly.

First, the latissimus dorsi muscle is sutured inferiorly, approximately 2 to 3 cm below the submammary line, with interrupted fine nylon su-tures. Then it is sutured superiorly, without tension to the undersurface of the pectoralis major muscle. Using temporary silicone implant sizers, the appropriate size of the implant may be determined, as well as the necessary tension under which the muscle will be sutured superiorly and inferiorly while allowing a safe skin closure. The pocket is closed laterally and superiorly by anchoring the lateral edge of the latissimus dorsi muscle to the serratus musculature with several sutures, and by approximating the latissimus dorsi muscle to the lateral edge of the sternum *(Fig. 3.7)*. If there is not sufficient muscle beyond the inferior edge of the skin island to suture it to the chest wall below the inframammary line, the edge of the latissimus dorsi muscle is sutured to the undersurface of the inferior chest skin flap so as to provide an adequate pocket that will accept the implant.

Sutures are placed (but not tied) inferiorly and laterally to allow insertion of a prosthesis *(Fig. 3.8)*. Sutures are then tied, and if additional ones

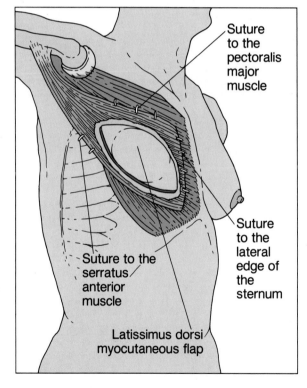

Suture to the pectoralis major muscle

Suture to the lateral edge of the sternum

Suture to the serratus anterior muscle

Latissimus dorsi myocutaneous flap

FIG. 3.7

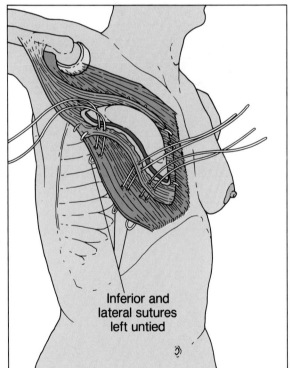

Inferior and lateral sutures left untied

FIG. 3.8

are needed, they are placed carefully to avoid puncturing the prosthesis *(Fig. 3.9)*.

Finally, the skin island is adjusted and positioned with temporary staples to orient and tailor it accordingly. When one is satisfied with the appropriate projection and shape, final closure is performed with subcuticular sutures of fine nylon *(Figs. 3.10, 3.11)*. Only dermal approximation is necessary. The inferior tip of the skin island usually is rounded off, and any excess skin at the superior end of the skin island is resected leaving the subcutaneous tissue to simulate the axillary tail of the breast. An additional drain may be placed along the axillary dissection, but no drains are placed along the reconstructive implant itself.

The patient is then dressed with a circumferential figure 8 bandaging which pushes the prosthesis medially and inferiorly.

Specific Considerations

Donor Site

When the back serves as the donor site for the skin island, the skin may be positioned anywhere over the surface of the latissimus dorsi muscle. The skin island may be transverse, oblique, or midoblique.

TRANSVERSE DESIGN. If the skin island is oriented transversely, just below the tip of the scapula, it will be closed with a straight line scar (easily covered by a brassiere and much preferred by the patients). This places the skin island at the superior border of the latissimus dorsi muscle, leaving the major extent of the muscle inferiorly. As one transposes the island to the chest wall, most of the muscle will be located superiorly and will reach the subclavicular hollow. This method is,

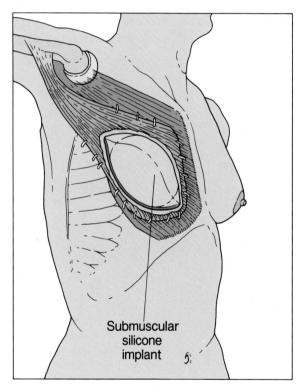

FIG. 3.9

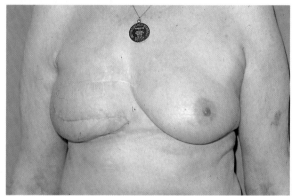

FIG. 3.10

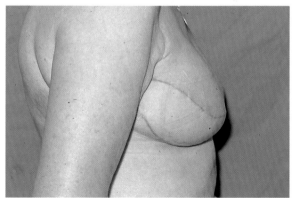

FIG. 3.11

Submuscular silicone implant

therefore, most appropriate for padding the subclavicular defect with muscle. The skin island, initially oriented transversely in the back, will now be oriented obliquely and should fit an oblique mastectomy scar *(Fig. 3.12.A)*.

OBLIQUE DESIGN. The skin island is oriented obliquely, just posterior to the anterior border of the latissimus dorsi muscle. It offers easy access to the free border of the muscle, which is readily found. The disadvantage of this design is that it offers little or no muscle above the transposed skin island; most of the muscle will lie inferiorly and laterally. Upon transposition, the skin island lies transversely *(Fig. 3.12.B)*.

MIDOBLIQUE DESIGN. A valuable compromise is found in the midoblique positioning of the skin island, because it offers the advantage of providing ample muscle both superiorly and inferiorly. The skin island can readily be positioned at the inframammary fold. The oblique scar in the back, however, is less desirable *(Fig. 3.12.C)*.

SHAPE OF THE SKIN ISLAND. Traditionally, the skin island has been drawn as an ellipse to facilitate closure of the donor site. An ellipse does not necessarily fulfill the requirements of reconstruction. The skin island can be placed anywhere on the latissimus dorsi muscle and designed in any shape or fashion. The most elegant skin island that offers advantages for reconstruction is that designed in a semilunar fashion with a central crescent *(see Fig. 3.25)*.

The semilunar arrangement has the advantage of simulating the inframammary fold, and the central crescent opens up the transverse diameter to provide more projection. The disadvantage of this arrangement is that the closure is not always obtained in a transverse line, and a small T-extension may be necessary. Regardless of the shape of the skin island, the donor site must be closed first and the use of skin grafts on the back must be avoided.

A helpful adjunct consists in drawing a pattern of the latissimus dorsi skin island and transposing it from the back to the chest, pivoting it at the approximate site of the thoracodorsal vessels. We have not made much use of this pattern because the skin islands do have some play, but we recommend it for the initial planning. Considering the amount of skin and muscle that can be obtained, donor site morbidity is minimal, other than seroma. To avoid the necessity of skin grafting on the back, the skin island should not be

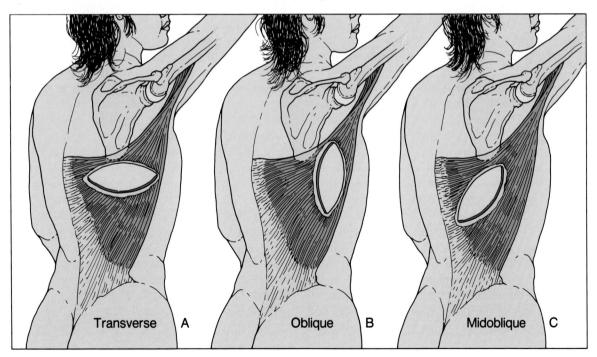

Transverse   A   Oblique   B   Midoblique   C

FIG. 3.12

wider than 7 to 8 cm. Beware of the common maneuver of determining the width of the skin island by pinching the excess skin with the fingers. The skin is under considerable tension and, once that tension is released, what appeared to be an easy closure may become excessively tight or impossible.

Over the long term, approximately 6 months to 1 year, there is no functional deficit from the transposition of the latissimus dorsi muscle. A flattening on the back, as well as a minimal asymmetry and winging of the scapula on the affected side are noticed.

Recipient Site

The variety of mastectomy scars facing the reconstructive surgeon poses a dilemma about flap placement. Scars can be vertical, transverse, or oblique. The temptation exists to excise the existing scar and to fit the flap to the defect. Experience has shown, however, that this approach does not always meet the objectives of reconstruction.

If the mastectomy has been performed through a transverse scar, one should note that this scar is now higher than desired. If one were to place the skin island at this place, the result usually would be unsatisfactory because one would have to fix the inframammary fold at a lower level from the skin island. Also, the color and texture of skin from the back is different from that of the chest skin and would be noticeable in a low-cut dress. Furthermore, there will be no increase in skin for projection, because the transverse diameter from midsternum to the midaxillary line has not been increased. Thus, placing the skin island transversely over a transverse scar is not recommended, except in rare occasions.

The best results are obtained by placing a skin island, which may be semilunar or in the form of a lazy S, in such a way that the vertical component lies along the anterior axillary line. The transverse component is placed at the inframammary line.

An additional maneuver that may be helpful in increasing the transverse diameter to give more projection is to do a Z-plasty at the level of the transverse mastectomy scar. This should be attempted only if the tissue is of good quality and has not been irradiated. This maneuver also corrects a transverse depression over the implant due to the underlying scarring of the skin and muscle. However, it should not be done if there is any question about the quality of the skin flaps.

The additional scars on the chest as well as on the back are a reasonable price if a naturally shaped and symmetric breast is obtained. On the other hand, they can add to the distress of the patient and the surgeon if the result of the reconstructed breast is unsatisfactory.

The Implant

Usually some form of prosthetic implant must be used, but the choice of a device that contains gel, saline or both is an individual one. An inflatable implant has the advantage of allowing intraoperative volume adjustment, but there is an increased risk of leakage.

Most implants continue to be plagued with the problems of capsular formation. What initially appears to be a soft and pliable breast reconstruction may become a firm and spherical one due to capsular contraction. If implants are placed 2 to 3 cm below the opposite inframammary fold, compensation for the inevitable capsular contraction will be achieved.

The use of the combination gel and saline implants has a temporary advantage in that the size can be adjusted more easily. We use a gel implant particularly if the proper size has been determined with the use of a "sizer" implant.

The implant is placed with its upper portion covered by the pectoralis major muscle and, in most cases, the inferior portion by the latissimus dorsi muscle. No attempt is made to cover the implant entirely with a combination of pectoralis and serratus anterior muscles. Similarly, one is always cautious of placing the implant too high, because it is impossible to bring it down in the postoperative period. Conversely, proper taping may bring up a somewhat lower implant. The size of the implant must conform not only to the needs of the reconstruction, but also to the dictates of flap tension. Inevitable flap edema in the postoperative period increases tissue tension and may disrupt the wound. On the other hand, in every case, the implant is placed at the same sitting, and moderate tension does not affect the viability of the flap.

Specific Problems

A considerable number of mastectomy patients show some atrophy of the pectoralis major muscle. This is due to an injury of the lateral or medial pectoral nerves which may occur as the surgeon retracts or divides the pectoralis minor muscle to reach the apex of the axilla. This results in atrophy of the inferior lateral half of the pectoralis major muscle.

In addition, in most patients the breast tissue itself has a takeoff at a certain distance below the clavicle. Because the takeoff is higher in some women, a hollow may be present in that area which is most annoying to the patients because it cannot be covered with clothes. The hollow in the upper chest has not been adequately addressed or corrected. Using patterned silicone implants has produced only temporary improvement because they usually form a capsule and the borders are noted. The custom implant usually drops and ends up being removed.

Dermal grafts offer a partial solution. An additional partial solution is to change the suturing of the upper portion of the latissimus dorsi muscle. Rather than suturing underneath the pectoralis major muscle, one can do so over the muscle and to the undersurface of the skin flap. This will give a partial correction of the upper chest concavity.

Irradiation of the Chest Wall

Postmastectomy patients who have received preoperative or postoperative radiation to the chest wall and axilla present an increased risk for skin slough and wound healing problems. The skin and scar of the anterior chest wall should be carefully examined for evidence of telangiectasia, dermal and subcutaneous atrophy, brawny edema, and in some cases subcutaneous fibrosis.

Reconstruction is not contraindicated in irradiated patients if the latissimus dorsi flap used is very healthy. Using the flap may actually be advantageous. However, irradiated skin is best excised if damage is considerable. The skin flap should be elevated at a minimum, and if possible at the submuscular plane. If an implant is used (which we do not recommend), it must be covered in its entirety with muscle. This way, if the irradiated skin disrupts, the implant will be protected by the muscle layer. There is a greater chance for more severe capsular contracture in postradiated patients, but the latissimus dorsi myocutaneous flap is quite safe.

Clinical Cases

CASE 1.   Figures 3.13, 3.14 show a 50-year-old patient who had a radical mastectomy. The ten-

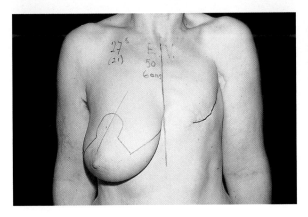

FIG. 3.13

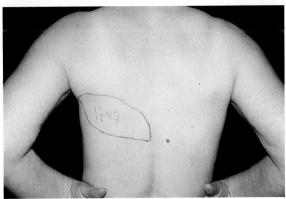

FIG. 3.14

don of the latissimus was transferred to the anterior surface of the humerus to simulate the tendon of the pectoralis muscle *(Fig. 3.15)*. The implant was introduced before closure of the breast pocket *(Fig. 3.16)*.

Figure 3.17 shows the patient 2 months later, before nipple-areola work and additional correction of the right breast. Six months later, symmetry is satisfactory and the breast is soft, but the areola of upper thigh skin remains too dark *(Figs. 3.18–3.21)*. The long donor scar is stretched and only partly hidden under the brassiere *(Fig. 3.22)*.

CASE 2. *Figures 3.23, 3.24* show the preoperative state of a 45-year-old patient 9 months after mastectomy. The indication for the flap reconstruction is the need to create a large breast for symmetry.

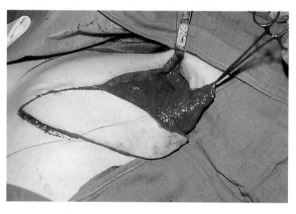

FIG. 3.15

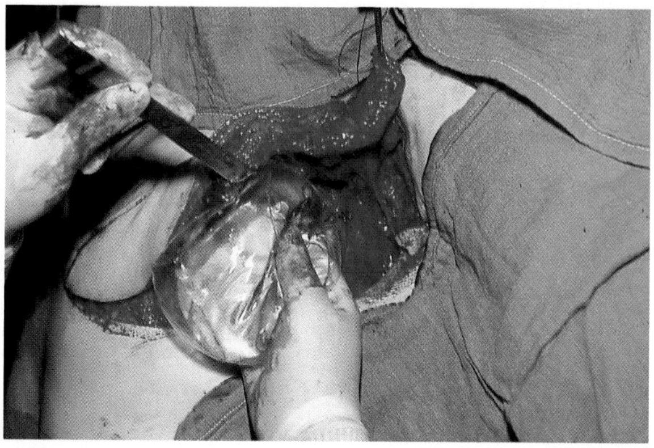

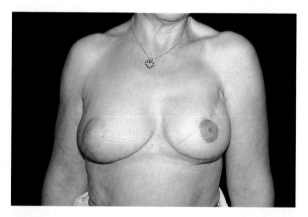

FIG. 3.16

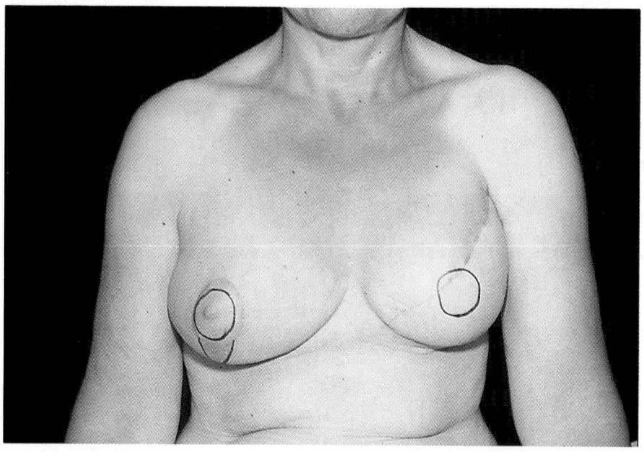

FIG. 3.17

FIG. 3.18

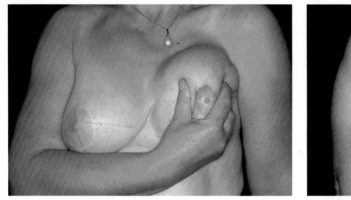

FIG. 3.19

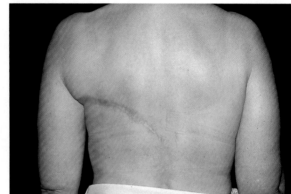

FIG. 3.20

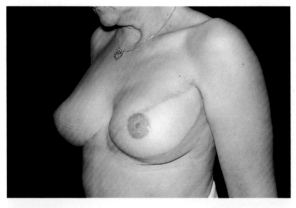

FIG. 3.21

FIG. 3.22

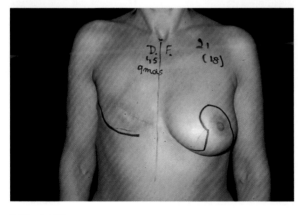

FIG. 3.23

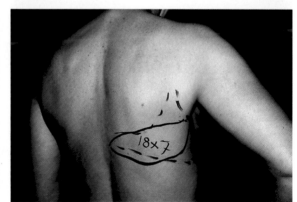

FIG. 3.24

Figures 3.25–3.27 show the patient 2 months later, before areola reconstruction. The implant is easily dislocated to the back. This complication can be prevented by making only a small, high tunnel in the axilla and avoiding a large communication of the chest and back wound. The pocket will be closed during nipple-areola reconstruction. *Figure 3.28* (following page) shows the patient 5 months later, and *Figures 3.29–3.31* show her 9 months after surgery.

RECONSTRUCTION OF BOTH BREASTS WITH BILATERAL LATISSIMUS DORSI MYOCUTANEOUS FLAPS

On occasion it may be desirable to reconstruct both breasts simultaneously with bilateral latissimus dorsi island myocutaneous flaps. Asymmetry for this procedure is lessened, particularly if the mastectomies were similar. Bilateral latissimus dorsi myocutaneous flaps are indicated in patients with subcutaneous mastectomy who have undergone a multitude of operations and who present with implant exposure and ulceration. The procedure is also applicable to patients with irradiated skin and to those who have very tight skin over the chest or have undergone extensive mastectomies. Some of these same patients are also candidates for the TRAM flap. Clinical judgment should be exercised for the application of the appropriate procedure.

Preoperative Planning

In the preoperative planning, determination is made whether the mastectomies have been symmetric and equal *(Figs. 3.32, 3.33)*. One may have been a modified mastectomy and the other one a simple mastectomy, in which the skin requirements will be different. The location of the mastectomy scars is noted, and the placement of the

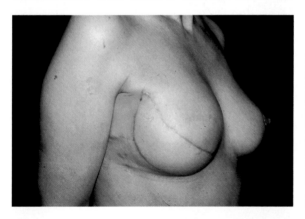

FIG. 3.25

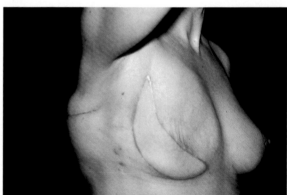

FIG. 3.26

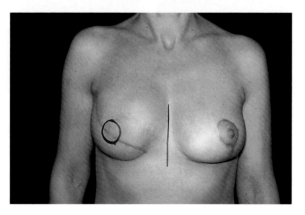

FIG. 3.27

latissimus dorsi skin islands is determined. It is important to locate the inframammary folds symmetrically on both sides and to decide on the shape of the latissimus dorsi skin islands as well as their position in the back.

Surgical Technique

The patient is positioned prone on the operating table and, if possible, two teams work simultaneously. The skin islands have been marked pre-

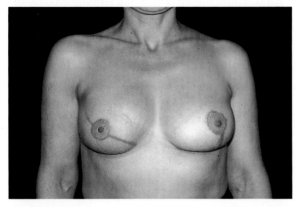

FIG. 3.28

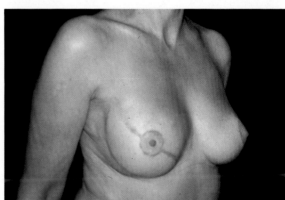

FIG. 3.29

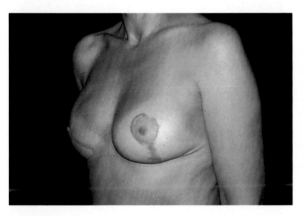

FIG. 3.30

FIG. 3.31

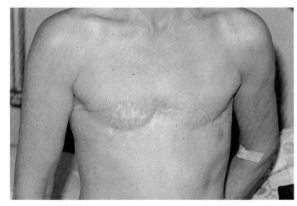

FIG. 3.32

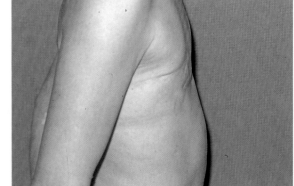

FIG. 3.33

operatively for shape and location. The myocutaneous flaps are then elevated simultaneously making sure that no excessive blood loss occurs (as discussed in the previous Surgical Technique). The elevation extends and is directed toward the axilla, particularly freeing the muscle from its posterior attachment along the tip of the scapula *(Fig. 3.34)*.

Once the flaps are elevated bilaterally, they are enclosed in a sterile plastic bag. If there is sufficient space in the axilla, they are packed there to be re-

trieved later when the patient is turned. The back wound is closed in layers with fine nylon, and a suction catheter is brought out through the lower edge of the incision *(Fig. 3.35)*.

The patient is then turned supine and redraped. Two operating teams can work simultaneously on the anterior chest. The principal surgeon directs the symmetry and the requirements of each type of mastectomy.

The myocutaneous flaps are placed over the

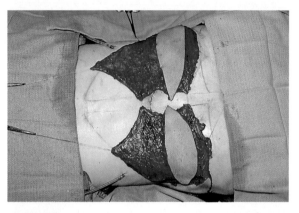

FIG. 3.34

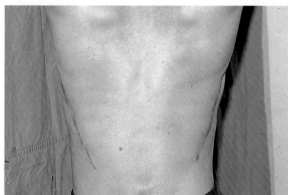

FIG. 3.35

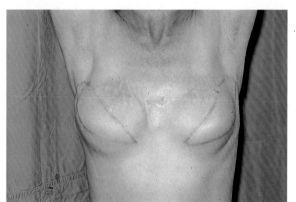

FIG. 3.36

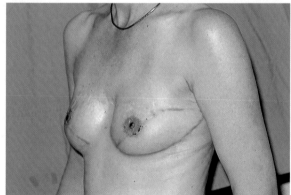

FIG. 3.37

chest and a determination is made as to the type of incisions to be made on each side. The objective is to form the inframammary line with an extension along the anterior axillary line which provides excess skin to increase the transverse diameter *(Figs. 3.36, 3.37)*. The flaps are temporarily inset with staples, and implant sizers are used to check for symmetry. It is necessary to have the patient sit up as much as possible to make sure the inframammary folds are at the proper level and are symmetric. Symmetry is obtained, if necessary, with the use of different types of implant on each

side. Once symmetry is accomplished, the wounds are closed permanently.

Clinical Case

Figures 3.38, 3.39 show a 37-year-old patient with a modified radical mastectomy on the left side and a subcutaneous mastectomy on the right side. A bilateral latissimus flap was chosen, with an ellipse of skin for the left side only, for this thin patient. *Figures 3.40, 3.41* show the elevation of the flaps.

Five months later, the patient awaited nipple-

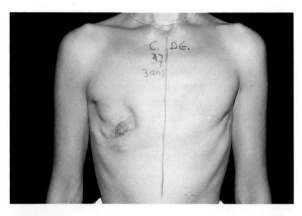

FIG. 3.38

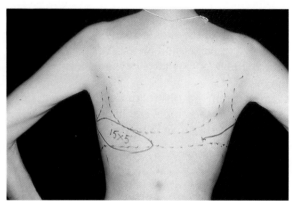

FIG. 3.39

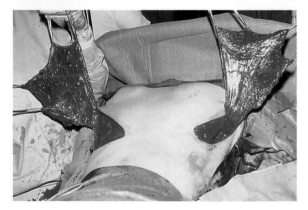

FIG. 3.40

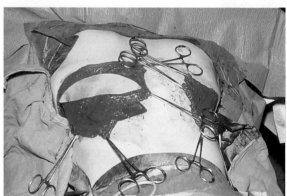

FIG. 3.41

areola reconstruction *(Fig. 3.42)*. The postreconstruction results are shown in *Figs. 3.43, 3.44.*

Two years later, the lack of subcutaneous tissue on the mastectomy side has become apparent *(Figs. 3.45, 3.46).*

Latissimus Reconstructions in Review

The safety of the method is exceptional and applies to all latissimus reconstructions. Only one flap was totally lost—at the beginning of our experience, when we were not aware of the risk of denervation and partial devascularization of the muscle by the mastectomy. Five flaps of 150 lost the distal tip of the skin island. This was probably due to excessive tension on the skin, or because the skin island was extended beyond the midline of the back.

In latissimus reconstructions, the second stage —creation of the nipple-areola complex—may be performed earlier than in other methods (i.e., after

2 months) because the shape of the breast is obtained earlier. Recent results have shown that the skin of the back takes on the aspect of the skin of the breast after several months, and the patchy appearance of the first months disappears unless the skin of the anterior chest has been damaged by the mastectomy or by radiotherapy.

The scar on the back has not been a problem, although it sometimes stretches and widens. No patient has complained of any functional disability after suppression of the muscle activity. It should be noted, however, that women undergoing this procedure were not athletic persons and the volume of their latissimus muscle is not to be compared with the muscular volume of women who are active in sports.

The percentage of capsular contractures—about 20% of grades III and IV—is higher than in simple reconstructions. This is probably related, in part, to the fact that flap reconstructions are performed in more complicated cases of mastectomy.

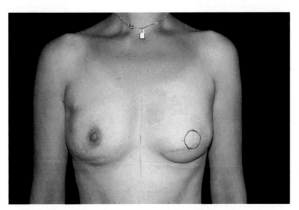

FIG. 3.42

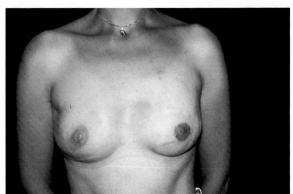

FIG. 3.43

FIG. 3.44

Another disappointing observation is the evolution of the muscle after transposition, although we always carefully preserved its nerve and sutured it under some tension. In patients in whom another operation was indicated after several years, we have often noticed an atrophy of the muscular fibers, sometimes so severe that muscle was hardly detectable. Pressure from the implant undoubtedly adds to muscle atrophy.

It should therefore be accepted that the thick muscular cover placed over the whole surface of the implant is temporary and may only prevent immediate complications. In our experience, the muscle fibers often retract from their distal position, no matter how careful the suturing may have been. This is shown during muscular contraction. In some recent cases, the coverage over the medial and lower parts of the breast was so thin that a few extrusions of the implant resulted. In these cases, the margins of the ulcer showed no muscular fibers at all.

A common unpleasant consequence of latissimus reconstructions are upward and lateral movements of the areola by adduction of the arm, which sometimes also produces wrinkling of the breast skin. Curiously, this has never been of any concern for our patients; they demonstrated it only when they were asked.

On the whole, satisfactory results have been obtained in the majority of cases of latissimus reconstruction. The major drawback of the method is, as in simple implantation, the rate of severe capsular contractures.

REVISION OF BREAST RECONSTRUCTION WITH A LATISSIMUS DORSI MYOCUTANEOUS FLAP

A common occurrence in reconstruction of the breast with a latissimus dorsi procedure is that the unit is almost never completely freed by dividing the attachments along the level of the tip of the scapula all the way toward its insertion on the humerus. Freeing this unit superiorly is relatively easy and bloodless, as long as one maintains and protects the neurovascular bundle. In this fashion, the unit is transposed as a pendulum and not by a rotational maneuver. If one does not free the unit completely, the pivot point will be along the posterior axillary line and the skin island will not reach the medial aspect of the chest. In addition, a bothersome bulge will occur along the axilla. Division of the insertion of the latissimus dorsi is not necessary, because it does not interfere with its transposition as a pendulum.

Clinical Case

The patient, a 56-year-old woman, had undergone a right modified mastectomy for carcinoma of the breast. All axillary nodes were negative, and the patient did not receive chemotherapy or radiotherapy. A breast reconstruction was performed using the latissimus dorsi myocutaneous flap. Following the procedure, the patient and the physician were displeased with the result.

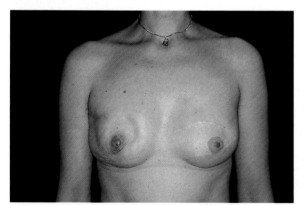

FIG. 3.45

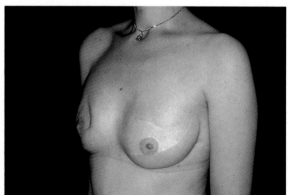

FIG. 3.46

Figure 3.47 demonstrates the reconstructed right breast, which does not match the opposite, slightly ptotic, teardrop-shaped breast. The inframammary fold is not well demarcated or symmetric with the opposite side, and there is a bulge along the axillary fold. The skin island of the latissimus dorsi has been inset through a separate scar disregarding the mastectomy scar. *Figure 3.48* shows a lack of fullness at the beginning of the inframammary fold near the sternum, and the bothersome bulging at the midaxillary line.

Evaluation of this patient indicated that the fault of the reconstruction was due to an inadequate transposition of the latissimus flap. The skin island was not placed in the parasternal area corresponding to the beginning of the inframammary line of the contralateral breast. Its correction ne-

cessitated redoing the operation and freeing the latissimus unit completely, leaving it attached only by its vascular pedicle and insertion along the humerus. Then the island of skin could be reinserted at the proper level.

In transposing the latissimus dorsi unit from the back to the chest, it is imperative to free the posterosuperior aspect of the muscle, particularly along the scapula and toward the axilla, leaving the unit attached only by the neurovascular pedicle and its insertion along the humerus. Once freed, the myocutaneous unit will transpose as a pendulum and will be ready to be inset at the proper location.

If one fails to free the posterosuperior border of the latissimus dorsi muscle, the unit will act as a rotation flap, pivoting on the posterior attachment

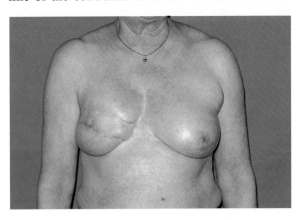

FIG. 3.47

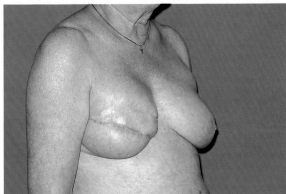

FIG. 3.48

instead of the thoracodorsal vessels and the tendinous insertion. This decreases the reach of the unit toward the chest and produces the bothersome bulge along the axilla.

Figure 3.49 shows the latissimus dorsi myocutaneous unit being freed posteriorly, reopening the previous scars and allowing the unit to swing like a pendulum only on its insertion and the vascular pedicle. A more pleasing contour and match of the ptotic effect with the contralateral breast were achieved *(Fig. 3.50).* The nipple had been placed relatively low to match appropriately the contralateral breast.

Figure 3.51 shows the correction of the bulging along the axillary line. Yet the persistence of the old mastectomy scar, with the additional incision corresponding to the placement of the latissimus skin island, is cause for concern.

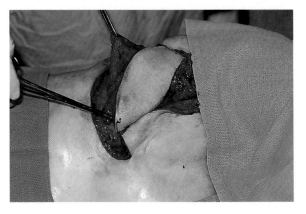

FIG. 3.49

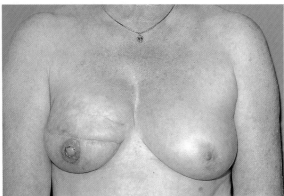

FIG. 3.50

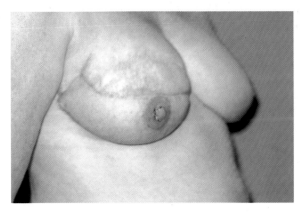

FIG. 3.51

CHAPTER·4

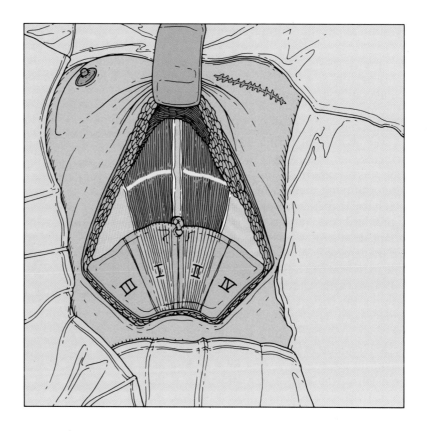

Breast Reconstruction with Flaps

LOWER TRANSVERSE RECTUS ABDOMINIS MUSCLE FLAP AND ABDOMINAL WALL CLOSURE

In the appropriate patient, the use of skin and subcutaneous tissue and fat from the infraumbilical area allows reconstruction of the breast without a silicone prothesis. Sufficient knowledge and clinical experience with this technique have been acquired to achieve symmetry, projection, and ptosis simulating the normal contour of the breast.[5]

The lower transverse rectus abdominis muscle (TRAM) flap *(Fig. 4.1)* differs from every other myocutaneous flap in that it is more tenuous and requires much more surgical respect. Complications such as necrosis of the flap and development of a lower abdominal hernia can be disastrous. Nevertheless, the versatility of the flap is such that it makes this procedure the most imaginative, lasting, and gratifying method of breast reconstruction. Clinical experience and anatomic studies have provided the various safeguards and the important details by which the safety of the procedure is increased. With proper execution, it is possible to reconstruct a symmetric breast with the patient's own tissue without the use of an implant. In addition, the patient obtains the benefits of an abdominoplasty. The long-term effects of this procedure have not been fully documented. The breast itself remains exactly as it is placed. The size and shape do not change, except for a slight gravitational fall of the soft tissues with time. If the abdominal wall is satisfactorily reconstructed, the loss of one or even both rectus muscles seems to be tolerated quite well by the patients. In the short term, there has been no noticeable weakness in the abdominal wall, no decreased exercise tolerance, and no disturbances of functions that require increased abdominal pressure, such as coughing, urination, or bowel movements.[5,7] Lordosis or scoliosis have not developed from the loss of balance of the abdominal musculature. Back pain, an early concern, has not been aggravated in patients who have undergone reconstruction of the breast with the TRAM flap.[4]

Anatomic Considerations

The flap is supplied by musculocutaneous perforating branches from the deep epigastric arcade that emerge in the periumbilical area *(Figs. 4.2, 4.3)*. Theoretically, a person needs to carry only a small amount of muscle—enough to preserve the deep epigastric arcade—and a narrow strip of fascia to include the two rows of periumbilical perforators. The flap may be adequately supplied by a minimum of one perforator, although this has not been studied. More perforators however are always desirable. Venous return is essential. The course of the blood is through the superficial epigastric veins

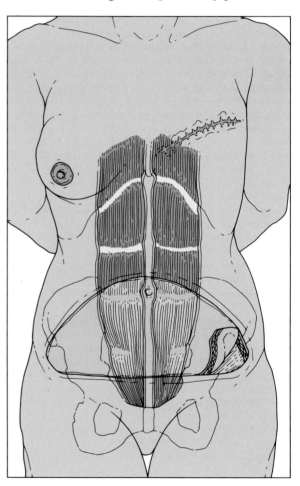

FIG. 4.1

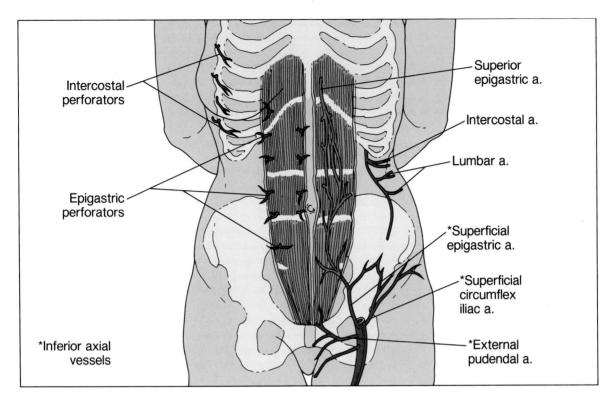

Intercostal
perforators

Epigastric
perforators

*Inferior axial
vessels

Superior
epigastric a.

Intercostal a.

Lumbar a.

*Superficial
epigastric a.

*Superficial
circumflex
iliac a.

*External
pudendal a.

FIG. 4.2

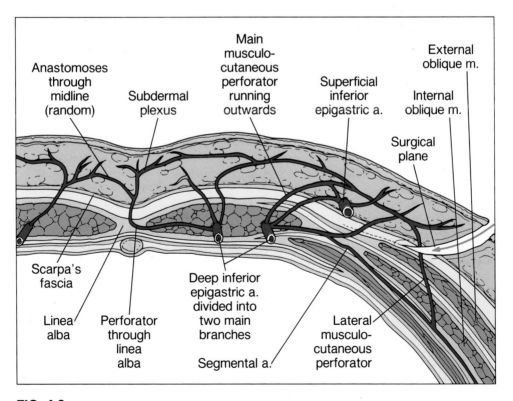

Anastomoses
through
midline
(random)

Subdermal
plexus

Main
musculo-
cutaneous
perforator
running
outwards

Superficial
inferior
epigastric a.

External
oblique m.

Internal
oblique m.

Surgical
plane

Scarpa's
fascia

Deep inferior
epigastric a.
divided into
two main
branches

Lateral
musculo-
cutaneous
perforator

Linea
alba

Perforator
through
linea
alba

Segmental a.

FIG. 4.3

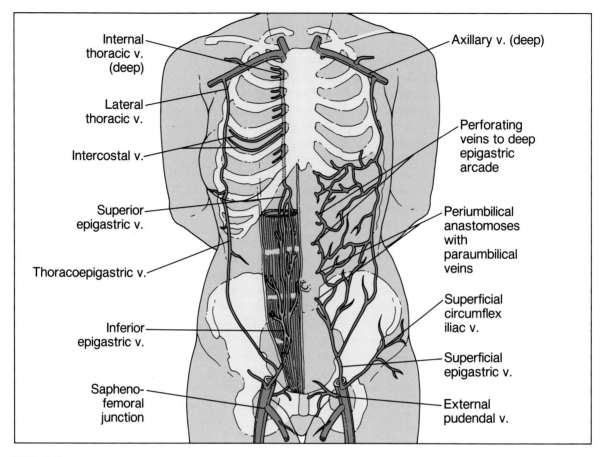

Internal thoracic v. (deep)

Lateral thoracic v.

Intercostal v.

Superior epigastric v.

Thoracoepigastric v.

Inferior epigastric v.

Sapheno-femoral junction

Axillary v. (deep)

Perforating veins to deep epigastric arcade

Periumbilical anastomoses with paraumbilical veins

Superficial circumflex iliac v.

Superficial epigastric v.

External pudendal v.

FIG. 4.4

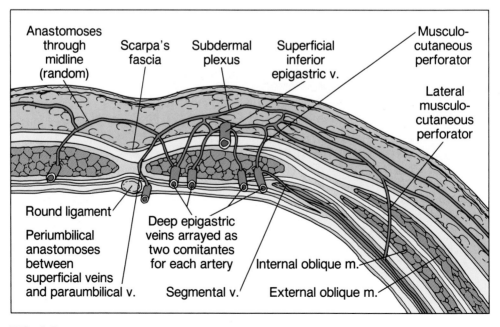

Anastomoses through midline (random)

Scarpa's fascia

Subdermal plexus

Superficial inferior epigastric v.

Musculo-cutaneous perforator

Lateral musculo-cutaneous perforator

Round ligament

Periumbilical anastomoses between superficial veins and paraumbilical v.

Deep epigastric veins arrayed as two comitantes for each artery

Segmental v.

Internal oblique m.

External oblique m.

FIG. 4.5

located just above Scarpa's fascia. These veins then perforate the fascia and eventually join the venae comitantes of the deep inferior epigastric artery *(Figs. 4.4, 4.5)*.

Valves that help overcome the effect of gravity have been observed in the deep venae comitantes.[2] For this reason, the flap has a tendency to become blue when left dependent on the inferior abdomen. The color improves as it is brought up to the chest and the venous return is facilitated.

Preservation of the Deep Epigastric Arcade

The deep epigastric arcade must be preserved by including that portion of the muscle in the flap *(Fig. 4.6)*. The arcade is located in the lateral third of the muscle; it is advisable for the surgeon to identify the arcade inferiorly at the point where the deep inferior epigastric artery enters the muscle.

Thus, the most lateral portion of the rectus abdominis may be preserved. In practice, only rarely do we preserve 2 to 3 cm of the lateral edge of the rectus muscle, which may not remain functional because its innervation has been divided.[3] It is easier to preserve the medial portion of the muscle in the infraumbilical area, but care must be exercised as the dissection is extended toward the xiphoid, where the entrance of the superior epigastric artery is variable. The medial portion of the muscle will be denervated and will not be functional. In most cases, the medial portion of the muscle is not spared. Presently, we advise including the entire rectus muscle with the flap.

The important perforators are located in the periumbilical area. The surgeon may transect the muscle at the level of the semicircular line, preserving the pyramidal muscle. Anchoring the dis-

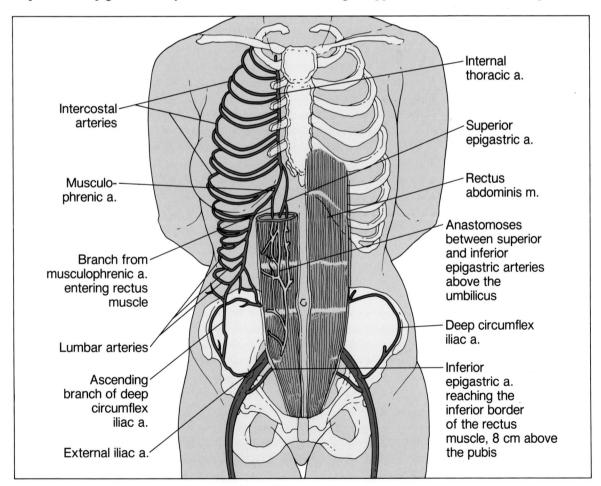

Intercostal arteries

Musculo-phrenic a.

Branch from musculophrenic a. entering rectus muscle

Lumbar arteries

Ascending branch of deep circumflex iliac a.

External iliac a.

Internal thoracic a.

Superior epigastric a.

Rectus abdominis m.

Anastomoses between superior and inferior epigastric arteries above the umbilicus

Deep circumflex iliac a.

Inferior epigastric a. reaching the inferior border of the rectus muscle, 8 cm above the pubis

FIG. 4.6

tal end of the rectus abdominis muscle to the medial and lateral remnants of the rectus fascia and to the semicircular line helps prevent the bulging that occurs if the muscle is removed or allowed to retract below the semicircular line.

Preservation of the Anterior Rectus Fascia

It is essential to preserve a segment of fascia on either side of the perforating vessels from the epigastric arcade.[4] This is easily achieved, because the line of perforators is located 2 to 3 cm lateral to the midline. A 3- to 4-cm segment of fascia is included throughout the length of the rectus muscle from the origin of the muscle, along the costal margin, to the lower edge of the skin flap below the semicircular line. Because there are only a few perforators inferior to the semicircular line, the surgeon can save enough fascia to effect a direct closure without the use of prosthetic materials.

A helpful safeguard in the operative procedure requires elevating the upper abdominal flap first to the costal margin, noting the row of perforators with hemoclips or electrocautery. The segment of fascia is then outlined, so as to preserve as much midline and lateral fascia as possible. An additional safeguard is, next, to elevate the "random" side of the flap, noticing again the row of perforators. The flap side with the muscle and vascular pedicle is elevated last.

Contralateral or Ipsilateral Use of Muscle

Using the rectus abdominis muscle contralateral to the side being reconstructed makes rotation of the flap easier. One does not need to twist the pedicle more than 90° *(Fig. 4.7.A).*[1] The rotation and twist are smooth, tension-free, and do not seem to interfere with the venous return. They also allow safe shaping of the breast.

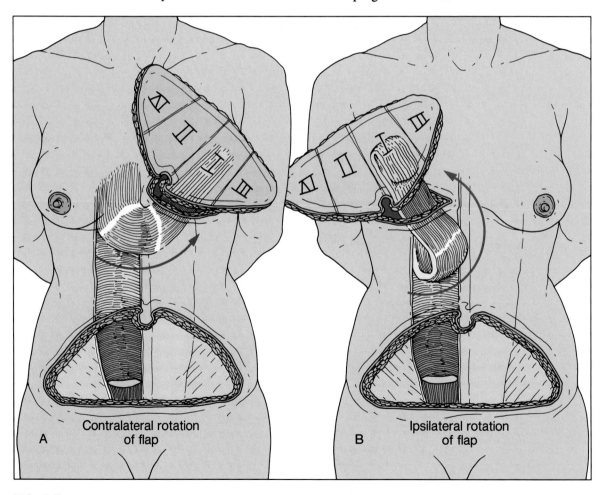

A   Contralateral rotation of flap

B   Ipsilateral rotation of flap

FIG. 4.7

Dissection is no more difficult on the ipsilateral side than on the contralateral side, and the reach of the flap is shorter. Some problems do occur because the flap requires at least a 270° twist to keep the skin to the outside and to obtain a satisfactory shaping of the breast *(Fig. 4.7.B)*.

In both cases, the site of the umbilicus on the flap serves as a guide for an initial anchoring of the flap and for the proper shaping of the breast.

Location of Flap (High or Low) in Trunk

The flap must be marked on the abdomen at the level of the umbilicus, because the important perforators are at the periumbilical area *(Fig. 4.8)*. Placing the flap any higher than this is not advantageous and has the drawback of shortening the arc of rotation, thus requiring further superior dissection of the flap to reach the chest. The inferior incision should be placed at the level at which a primary closure can be accomplished without excessive tension. In almost all cases, it falls at the same level as in an aesthetic abdominoplasty. To obtain a symmetric infraabdominal scar, the surgeon should tailor the final closure to achieve a straight horizontal scar of equal bilateral length. Only in the case of unacceptable and multiple infraumbilical scars which may affect the blood supply is the flap outlined above the umbilicus. Obesity, lower midline, or Pfannenstiel-type incisions have not precluded using a low design at the umbilical level.

Location of Inframammary Fold

In every method of breast reconstruction, re-creation of the inframammary fold is essential. Its placement is determined from the contralateral side. The surgeon should keep in mind, however, that there may be an inferior pull on the upper

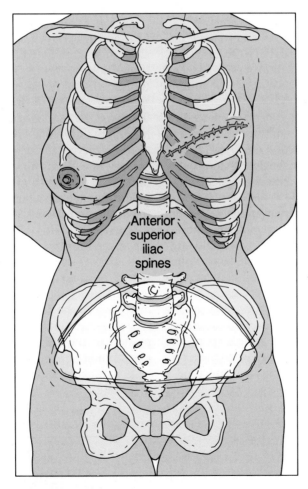

Anterior superior iliac spines

FIG. 4.8

abdominal flap and a slight but definite pull from the rectus abdominis muscle, as well as the effect of gravity.

Consequently, it is advised that a portion of the inframammary fold be left intact and undisturbed by the dissection. The surgeon must not connect the abdominal dissection with the chest dissection, except by a high tunnel wide enough to accommodate the passing of the flap. Placing the TRAM flap too low or too high detracts from the aesthetic result of the reconstruction. However, it is easier to correct a flap placed too low by raising the inframammary line, than the reverse.

Selection of Patients

When using autogenous tissue for breast reconstruction, the surgeon avoids the major cause of secondary problems and disappointment: the breast implant. Abdominal tissue is the only sufficient and satisfactory source of replacement for an amputated breast, because it does not create distortion and asymmetry as does the gluteal free flap. Moreover, in most cases, it improves the general aspect of the patient by producing a "tummy tuck" effect.

This operation, however, is a major procedure which requires several prerequisites. The patient should be in good condition and motivated for the reconstruction. She must understand that recovery after this kind of operation takes 4 to 6 weeks, and that there is a risk of complications.

Even if the patient is strongly motivated, there are some absolute and relative contraindications for this method. Some are related to general conditions, such as bad prognosis of the cancer, poor general health, hypertension, diabetes, arteriosclerosis, excessive obesity, smoking habits, and/or psychological imbalance. Other contraindications are related to local conditions—excessive thinness, insufficient abdominal skin, multiple scars on the upper or lower abdomen, and damage to the internal mammary artery by irradiation or surgery.

Only experience can help the surgeon in judging the importance of all these factors and deciding if the method is totally contraindicated or if it can be adapted. For instance, in some high-risk cases, it may be advisable to take a double rectus pedicle or to place the flap higher on the abdomen to include more perforators.

Preoperative Evaluation of the Patient

Appropriate patients for the TRAM flap procedure are women who have had children and, as a result, often have some excess skin in the lower abdomen that makes them good candidates for an abdominoplasty. This type of reconstruction has been performed, however, on nulliparous women, usually older than 35 years, with a slightly convex abdomen.

A preoperative decision is made as to whether the opposite breast is to be matched, thereby taking appropriate measurements, locating the inframammary line, and planning for a normal projection and ptosis. Otherwise, to obtain symmetry one decides whether the opposite breast needs to be reduced or elevated (ptosis correction) which is done at the same time or during a second-stage procedure.

Appropriate measurements are taken with the patient standing to measure the deficit in the vertical and transverse diameter of the mastectomy site in comparison with the curved three-dimensional normal breast. The inframammary line is transposed to the flat mastectomy site, and measurements are taken from both the midclavicular line over the curved surface of the breast to the inframammary line, and from the midsternum over the curved surface of the breast to the anterior axillary line. This will determine the vertical and horizontal deficits *(Figs. 4.9–4.11)*.

The surgeon also marks the superior extent of the normal breast and determines the degree of the subclavicular hollow which needs to be filled with the de-epithelialized portion of the flap. The extension of the normal breast into the axillary fold should be compared with the deficit on the mastectomy site. Inspection also will reveal whether the contralateral breast is rounded or ptotic. The type of mastectomy scar will determine whether a portion of the chest skin (usually inferior to the scar) should be excised, or whether the flap should be de-epithelialized and placed at the inframammary line.

Pre- and Postoperative Care

Once it has been decided to use a TRAM flap, the patient is encouraged to exercise her abdominal wall regularly and to keep or obtain her ideal weight. She should stop smoking. This not only reduces the risk for the arterial input of the flap, but also avoids pulmonary complications caused by limited chest expansion, and fear of coughing after the operation. We do not prescribe any drugs before entry to the hospital, but the patient is prepared for autotransfusion by collection of 3 U of blood in the preoperative month.

In Belgium, the patient enters the hospital 2 days before the operation and undergoes a complete checkup, as well as bowel preparation by the oral route with 1 liter of polyethylene glycol. An IV is placed and the patient receives Zantac® the evening before the operation. This is not possible in the U.S., where the patient usually is admitted the night before or the morning of surgery.

Installation in the operating room takes approximately 1 hour. A peridural catheter, introduced to start sedation with Marcaine as soon as the operation is finished, is left in place during the first 2 or 3 days. Another option is the use of the self-administered analgesic machine, which delivers 1 to 2 mg of morphine every 15 minutes, as needed, for postoperative pain control.

The patient is positioned in a semisitting position on a heating blanket and the operating room is kept at a comfortable temperature. A stellate block is performed on the side of the flap to increase vasodilatation, if desired, but this is not essential. A venous pressure catheter and a bladder catheter are placed. Blood is replaced as needed, and fluids are given in sufficient amounts to maintain a normal venous pressure. During surgery, 500 mg of Solumedrol are administered.

After the operation, the patient remains in a semisitting position in a warm bed, with the flap adequately heated. She receives oxygen through a nasal catheter, 3 to 5 liters/min. Antibiotics are started preoperatively and are continued for 3 days.

The patient begins ambulation the day after the operation. During the first week, she is encouraged to walk without standing up straight. Postoperative transfusions are given if needed. Oral feedings are begun on restoration of bowel function. Abdominal distention is avoided. Recovery is usually rapid and patients return to a normal life within 4 to 6 weeks.

Pre- and postoperative care should be followed with maximal attention. Severe complications may result from errors in care, even if surgery has been adequate.

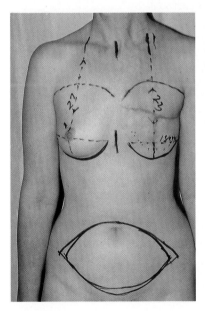

FIG. 4.9

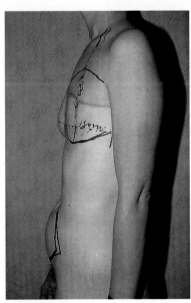

FIG. 4.10

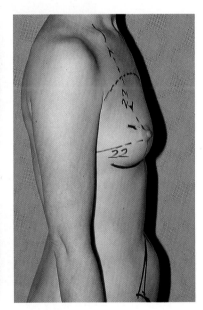

FIG. 4.11

Surgical Technique

Outline of the Flap

The flap is outlined with the upper incision placed at the umbilicus. The lower incision is made suprapubically as for an aesthetic abdominoplasty. It is placed at the level of the pubic hair, transverse up to a point directly below the anterior superior iliac spine on each side *(Fig. 4.12)*. From this point, the line takes a gentle 25° curve upward and extends as far laterally as necessary. Using the principle of triangulation, which places two sutures in the midline, one above the xiphoid and the second at the pubis, various points of this marking are transposed from one side to the other so that the flap is outlined symmetrically on both sides *(Fig. 4.13)*. The symmetric design allows a more aesthetically pleasing horizontal scar in the suprapubic area.

Whenever possible, the contralateral rectus abdominis muscle is used as a pedicle because of ease of rotation during reconstruction of the breast. As a teaching guide, the flap has been divided into fourths, each representing a numbered zone: zone I corresponds to the muscle ped-

icle; zone II, to the opposite rectus abdominis muscle; zone III, to the area of the flap lateral to the rectus abdominis muscle being raised; and zone IV, to the contralateral aspect of the flap *(Fig. 4.14)*. Obviously, zone IV is the most tenuous as far as blood supply is concerned and the one that is discarded in every case. Portions of zone II also may be discarded for the safety of the flap.

Elevation of the Flap

The umbilicus is first circumscribed by placing skin hooks at the 12 and 6 o'clock positions, and by making two straight vertical cuts. The hooks are then changed to the 3 and 9 o'clock positions, and two more straight incisions are made, usually circumscribing the umbilicus completely. The stalk of the umbilicus is then dissected down to the fascia.

The upper incision of the flap is made first; it is beveled at the periumbilical level, for approximately 3 cm from the midline and symmetrically on both sides, to preserve additional perforators. To preserve the superficial epigastric vessels, the beveling should be performed only to a level deep enough to reach Scarpa's fascia.

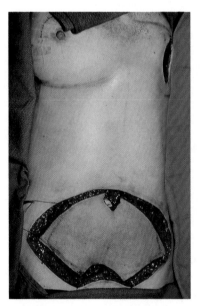

FIG. 4.12

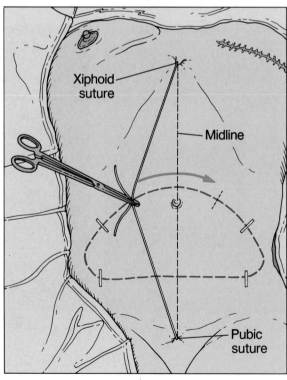

FIG. 4.13

The upper abdominal flap is elevated to the costal margin laterally, above the xiphoid medially, and superficial to the anterior rectus sheath. Whether the flap is ipsilateral or contralateral, a tunnel connecting with the chest incision should be high and on the contralateral side to avoid the bulge in the epigastrium from the muscle pedicle *(Fig. 4.15)*. If the contralateral muscle is used, the dissection of the chest skin is extended to the inframammary line but is not connected with the abdominal dissection. Preservation of these attachments ensures the correct delineation of the inframammary fold. As dissection of the upper abdominal flap is performed, two rows of perforators from the anterior rectus sheath, which must be divided, are encountered. These perforators will serve as a guide for the location of the important periumbilical perforators.

At this point, the segment of anterior rectus sheath to be included with the muscle is marked. This segment is usually 3 to 4 cm in width, and it should include the two rows of perforators. An incision is made on both sides of the fascia from above the costal margin to the upper level of the

abdominal flap. The medial and lateral aspects of the rectus abdominis muscle are then dissected out bluntly, except at the level of the intersectiones tendineae, where sharp dissection is needed. Leaving a segment of fascia over the entire length of the muscle is most advantageous because it facilitates freeing up the entire muscle.

Attention is now turned to the lower part of the flap. If unsure, the surgeon can test whether the upper flap will reach the lower incision at the pubic level by applying inferior traction and placing the patient in a sitting position. This maneuver often is unnecessary and not recommended in routine cases.

The lower incision is made by dividing completely across the superficial epigastric vessels on both sides down to the anterior rectus sheath and the external oblique fascia. The random side of the flap is elevated above the rectus fascia to approximately 1 cm beyond the midline. While performing this dissection, the surgeon should take note of the perforating vessels that are divided and pay particular attention to those at the periumbilical area. The lowermost perforator is marked, usually

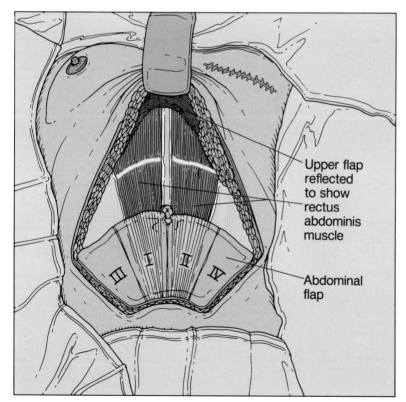

Upper flap reflected to show rectus abdominis muscle

Abdominal flap

FIG. 4.14

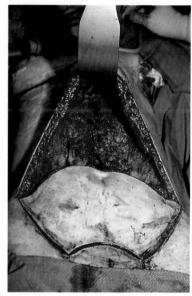

FIG. 4.15

at the level of the semicircular line. Small perforators near the midline also are divided. Although they are of little consequence to the flap *(Fig. 4.16.A)*, they may cause some anxiety.

The flap on the pedicle side is elevated rapidly to the lateral edge of the rectus abdominis muscle *(Fig. 4.16.B)*. Dissection is continued carefully to the point where the lateral fascial incision was made above the flap, so as to protect the row of perforators. By knowing the position of the rows of perforators superiorly and by preserving as much fascia as possible, 4 to 5 cm of fascia is included with the entire rectus muscle. This is sufficient to include the perforating vessels and, at the same time, to allow primary closure without the need for prosthetic mesh. The lateral edge of the fascia is carefully divided, and usually narrowed inferiorly near the pubis. Because the lateral incison is medial to the semilunar line, the layers are divided into the external and internal oblique fasciae which separate below the umbilicus.

The medial division of the fascia is done approximately 1 cm from the midline, using the superior fascia incision as a guide. The flap is gently retracted and the fascia is incised with either scissors or knife past the level of the lowest perforator, as determined from the opposite side. From this point on, the fascia is tapered into a triangle near the pubis.

Anchoring sutures placed between the anterior rectus fascia muscle and the skin flap do not help and are not essential; the attachments are quite secure without them. Following this approach, sufficient fascia is preserved for direct closure. Laterally, the important junction of the external oblique and anterior rectus fasciae is undisturbed, and 1 cm of fascia near the midline also is preserved.

Once the fascia is divided, the rectus muscle is freed bluntly, elevated anteriorly, and retracted medially. The deep inferior epigastric vessels are identified and divided between suture ligatures. Care must be exercised to ensure that the inferior epigastric vessels are included with the muscle and are not inadvertently left with the posterior rectus sheath. Medial and lateral segments of rectus abdominis muscle may be left to facilitate the closure *(Fig. 4.17)*.[4,5] Although we have at times preserved those segments of muscle up to the

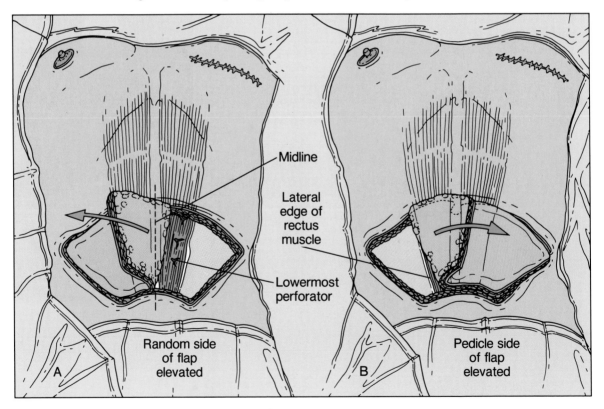

FIG. 4.16

umbilicus, we no longer do so, preferring to take the entire muscle. A decision to leave the lateral third of the muscle, if desired, should be made only after identifying the entrance of the inferior epigastric vessels. The entrance is variable and, on occasion, can be on the most lateral third of the muscle.

Because there is no posterior sheath below the semicircular line, it is a potential area of weakness. The muscle should be transected just below the semicircular line, preserving the remaining distal muscle to cover that weakened area and, thus, avoiding a lower abdominal bulge. Transection of the muscle at the level of the semicircular line is distressing, because the skin flap will be devoid of muscle in approximately its distal third. This is of no consequence, however, because the important perforators are above the semicircular line. The inclusion of muscle to the distal end of the skin flap is of no advantage.

The skin flap with the underlying rectus abdominis muscle is then dissected superiorly by freeing the muscle from the posterior rectus sheath and dividing the segmental intercostal vessels and nerves. The elevation extends all the way to the costal margin.

At this point, the surgeon should pause and remember that the superior epigastric vessels usually exit underneath the costal margin, approximately 2 to 4 cm lateral to the xiphoid.

Upon entering the muscle, the superior epigastric vessel divides into two branches that run medially and laterally. The dissection at the costal margin should be precise. If possible, the surgeon should identify the superior epigastric arcade vessel by Doppler, but this is not essential. In every case we divide the origin of the rectus abdominis muscle from the ribs by cutting the anterior rectus sheath as well as the muscle from the ribs above the costal margin. Dividing the muscle on the ribs is safe; in fact, an island can be made by dividing the distal and proximal insertions of muscle. The medial dissection of the rectus near the xiphoid, however, should be carried out with extreme care. The uppermost intercostal neurovascular bundle just below the costal margin is identified and at least the nerve is transected, so that the muscle will atrophy.

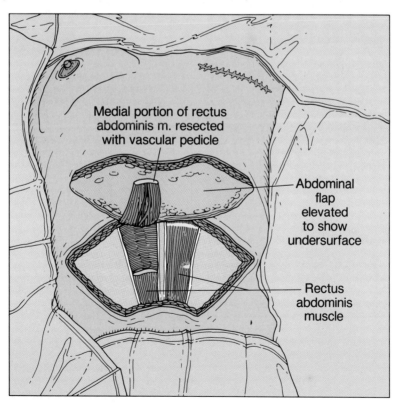

Medial portion of rectus abdominis m. resected with vascular pedicle

Abdominal flap elevated to show undersurface

Rectus abdominis muscle

FIG. 4.17

Reopening of the Mastectomy Scar

The mastectomy scar is now opened. A tunnel, extending almost to the contralateral breast, is created very high to connect with the abdominal incision on the contralateral side of the mastectomy. On the mastectomy side, the dissection is extended only to the level of the inframammary fold to preserve its attachments. The chest and the abdominal incisions on the mastectomy side should not be connected *(Fig. 4.18)*. The use of a suction-assisted lipectomy machine will facilitate removing some fat from the contralateral breast and upper abdomen. A tunnel of sufficient size to admit passage of the flap is made.

Passage of the Flap

The flap is thoroughly moistened with saline, and traction sutures are placed at the tips of zone IV. With the use of Deaver retractors, the skin flaps are elevated over the tunnel. The assistant applies gentle traction on the sutures while the surgeon pushes the flap toward the chest. The flap is then delivered to the chest. The orientation is such that zone IV will be superior, toward the axilla, while the umbilical area will lie at approximately the medial aspect of the inframammary line.

Shaping of the Breast

This is the primary and most challenging objective. Considerable time should be spent on this portion of the procedure, striving to match the opposite breast by using only the "safe" portions of the flap to achieve the proper level, projection, and ptosis. When the flap has been passed into the chest with zone IV oriented superiorly *(Fig. 4.19)*, there is a gentle 90° turn of the muscle pedicle which should not be tight. If this is not the case, the surgeon needs to free the muscle by cutting it

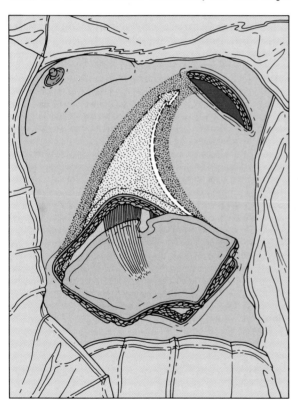

FIG. 4.18

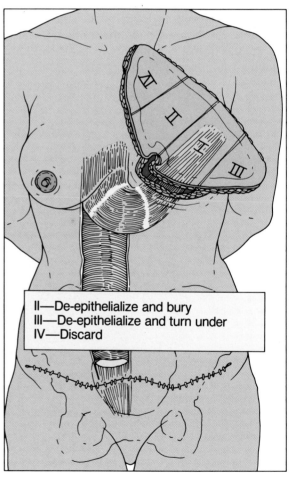

II—De-epithelialize and bury
III—De-epithelialize and turn under
IV—Discard

FIG. 4.19

on the ribs above the costal margin, thereby staying away from the superior epigastric vessels. The muscle pedicle is checked for a smooth and ample passage without extra kinks or excessive tension, and the color of the flap also is noted.

Zone IV and a portion of zone II are immediately discarded *(Figs. 4.20, 4.21)*. For purposes of molding, the site of the umbilicus is an excellent guideline. The umbilicus is to be placed at the medial border of the inframammary fold with a temporary suture or staple. Zone I will be placed along the inframammary line, and a decision is then made concerning excision or utilization of chest skin and de-epithelialization of the inferior portions of the TRAM flap. Excision of additional chest skin inferiorly usually is chosen, because this will hide the lower scar and decrease the "patch" appearance of the skin island.

Zone III, which is usually hanging down along the anterior axillary line, is to be de-epithelialized and tucked under. The inferior lateral location of the tissue of zone III is appropriate in that the breast volume is greater laterally and inferiorly. Temporarily shaping the breast with staples is most helpful. It should also be noted that, on re-opening the mastectomy scar, the upper skin flap is dissected superficially to the pectoralis major muscle up to the infraclavicular area, the inferior flap is dissected to the inframammary line, and both flaps are dissected laterally to the anterior

axillary line. The breast does not extend beyond these lines, and further dissection is unnecessary.

The shape of the new breast can be estimated by positioning the site of the umbilicus near the medial aspect of the inframammary line, placing the superior portion of the flap at the same level of takeoff of the breast superiorly, and situating zone III inferolaterally so it can be tucked under. This step is facilitated by the temporary use of staples. When the appropriate molding has been accomplished, it is worthwhile to place the patient in a sitting position (at least as much as possible) so that a comparison with the contralateral breast and final adjustments can be made. In general, the chest skin is excised to the inframammary line and the upper chest skin is broken with a zigzag incision to provide more projection.

Alternate Method of Molding the Breast
If one is sure of the viability of zone II or if a bilateral rectus flap has been done, a more conical and nicely shaped breast can be obtained by placing the umbilicus at 5 or 6 o'clock and allowing the flap to cone and project forward. On the other hand, this requires using portions of the entire zone II, which, if it were to necrose, would leave an unsightly scar on the parasternal area. We do not hesitate to use this alternative method of molding in patients younger than 45 years who seem to have healthier flaps.

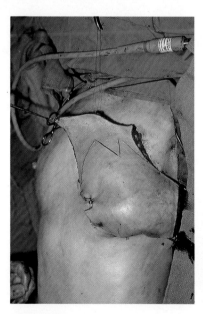

FIG. 4.20

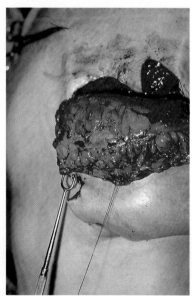

FIG. 4.21

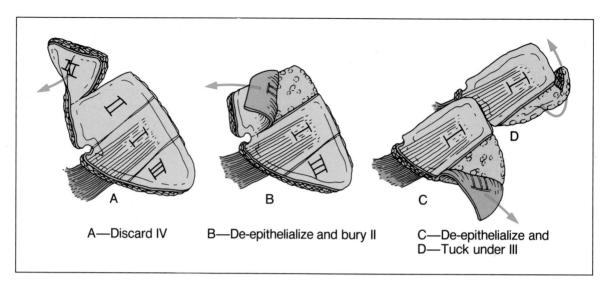

A—Discard IV   B—De-epithelialize and bury II

C—De-epithelialize and
D—Tuck under III

FIG. 4.22

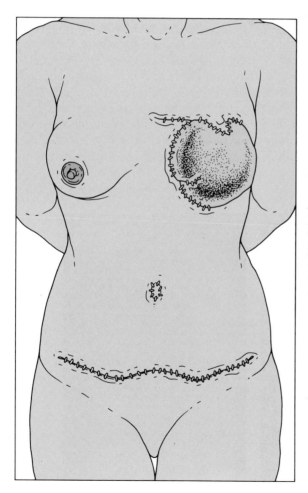

FIG. 4.23

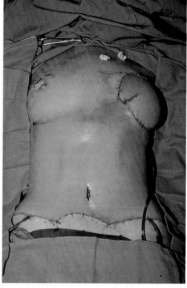

FIG. 4.24

De-Epithelialization of Upper and Inferior Lateral Portions of the Flap

With the temporary staples in place, the areas that need to be de-epithelialized can be marked *(Fig. 4.22)*. The de-epithelialization is performed at the dermal level with sharp dissection. It is usually a tedious procedure. Once this has been accomplished, it is necessary to hang the flap just above the line of takeoff of the breast to allow for some drooping due to gravity. Sutures are placed between the flap dermis and the pectoralis major muscle in a line that will extend to the axilla. If necessary, the proper de-epithelialization of a portion of the flap is performed to simulate the axillary tail. If the flap is quite thick, thinning is advisable by resecting the fat from the undersurface, below Scarpa's fascia.

Zone III is similarly marked and de-epithelialized so it can be tucked under. If the mastectomy scar has a transverse orientation, it is helpful to break the upper incision in a zigzag fashion to increase the horizontal diameter and to obtain more projection. An additional Z-plasty can be placed at the anterior axillary line. De-epithelialization is performed to correspond to the zigzag of the upper chest incision, and the upper end of the de-epithelialized flap is sutured to the pectoralis major muscle. Zone III is folded under and buried under zone *T* to give bulk and projection to the new breast. Zone IV is discarded.

Final Closure

The flap is supported in position with sutures fixed superiorly and medially. The skin edges are approximated either with fine nylon or in a subcuticular fashion.

While in the operating room, the patient should be placed in the sitting position so that breast symmetry can be checked. The newly reconstructed breast will not change and the final operative result is predictable and, in most cases, satisfying *(Figs. 4.23, 4.24)*. *Figures 4.25* and *4.26* show the early

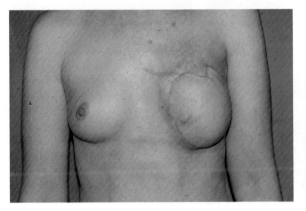

FIG. 4.25

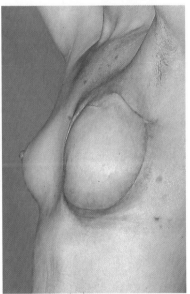

FIG. 4.26

postoperative result. *Figures 4.27–4.29* show the same patient with nipple-areola reconstruction.

Closure of the Abdominal Wall Following Unilateral and Bilateral Transverse Island Abdominal Flaps

Closure of the defect in the abdominal wall is begun immediately after the transverse island abdominal flap is delivered to the chest wall. A team of surgeons is molding the breast while another team proceeds with the abdominal closure. *Figures 4.30–4.32* show the defect in the abdominal wall following transfer of the unilateral and bilateral rectus muscle flaps.

In all cases, the rectus muscle has been transected at the level of the semicircular line and the upper border is reattached to the semicircular line with mattress sutures of nylon. This appears to strengthen the area where there is no posterior rec-

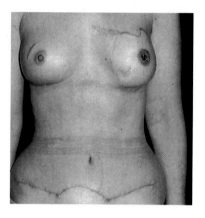

FIG. 4.27

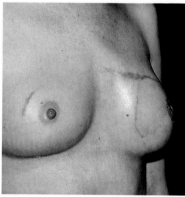

FIG. 4.28

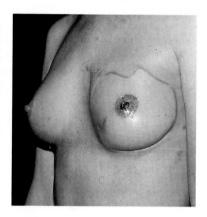

FIG. 4.29

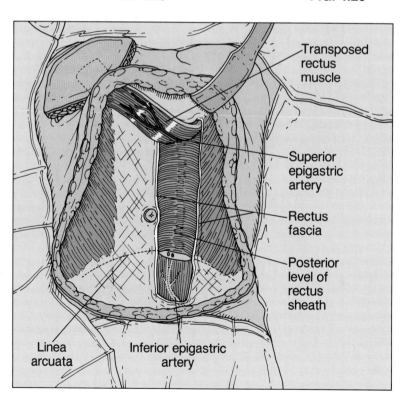

Transposed rectus muscle

Superior epigastric artery

Rectus fascia

Posterior level of rectus sheath

Linea arcuata

Inferior epigastric artery

FIG. 4.30

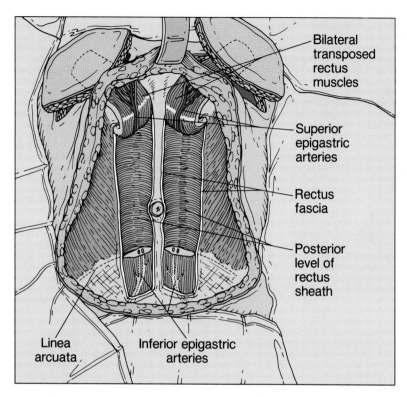

Bilateral
transposed
rectus
muscles

Superior
epigastric
arteries

Rectus
fascia

Posterior
level of
rectus
sheath

Linea
arcuata

Inferior epigastric
arteries

FIG. 4.31

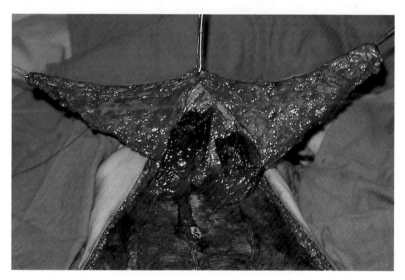

FIG. 4.32

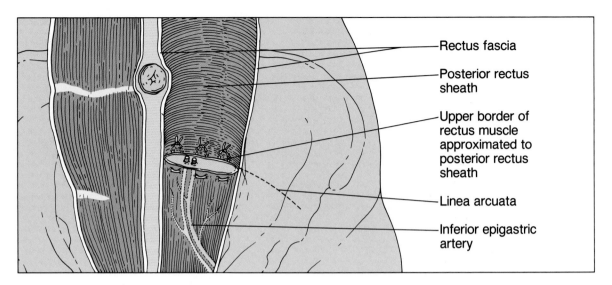

FIG. 4.33

- Rectus fascia
- Posterior rectus sheath
- Upper border of rectus muscle approximated to posterior rectus sheath
- Linea arcuata
- Inferior epigastric artery

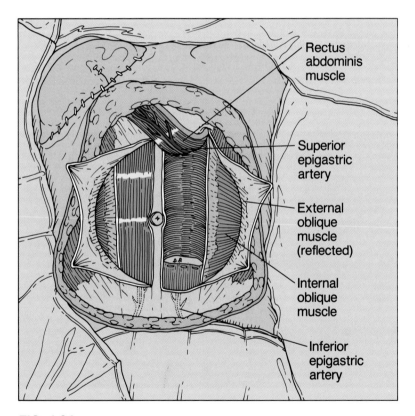

FIG. 4.34

- Rectus abdominis muscle
- Superior epigastric artery
- External oblique muscle (reflected)
- Internal oblique muscle
- Inferior epigastric artery

tus fascia, and prevents bulging as well as the pseudohernia in the suprapubic area *(Fig. 4.33)*.

The remnant of the anterior rectus sheath is then closed from its inferior extent to the level of the semicircular line. From this point on, the abdominal wall closure is accomplished by dissecting the external oblique fascia and muscle from the internal oblique one *(Figs. 4.34, 4.35)* and by doing a layered closure, bringing the internal oblique as close to the remnants of the midline rectus sheath as possible with interrupted sutures. The external oblique is approximated to the midline fascia as a separate layer on top of the internal oblique layer with running or interrupted sutures. This further reinforces the abdominal closure *(Figs. 4.36, 4.37)*. Care must be exercised in preserving the intercostal motor nerves *(Fig. 4.38)*.

In unilateral cases, closure of the anterior rectus sheath pulls the umbilical stalk toward the side of the closure. In addition, there is an apparent bulge on the normal side due to the flaccidity of the abdominal wall as well as the tightness and concavity from the removal of the rectus muscle. To correct this bulging, as well as any apparent flaccidity, the internal and external oblique muscles are advanced on the intact side. One begins by dividing the external oblique from the costal margin toward the inguinal ligament in a semilunar fashion just lateral to the rectus muscle. The external oblique musculoaponeurotic layer is freed toward the flanks (maintaining intact the underlying nerves as well as vessels) and is then advanced medially to be sutured to the anterior rectus sheath.

Before suturing the external oblique, the internal oblique muscle is plicated and sutured to the

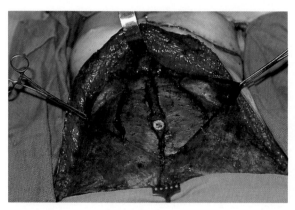

FIG. 4.35

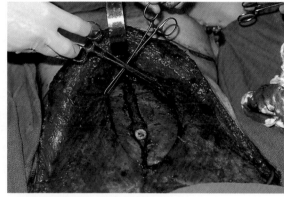

FIG. 4.36

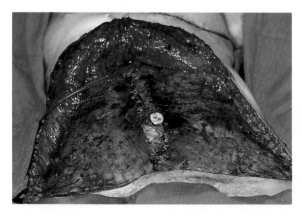

FIG. 4.37

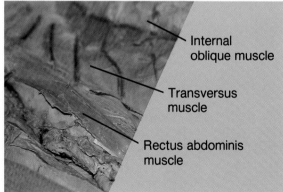

FIG. 4.38

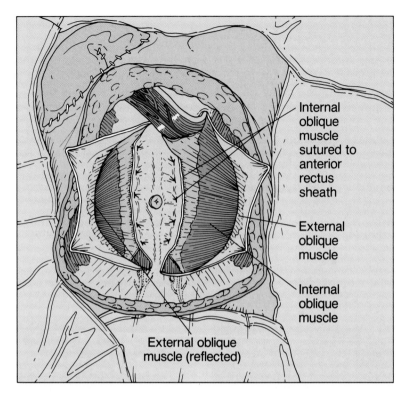

Internal oblique muscle sutured to anterior rectus sheath

External oblique muscle

Internal oblique muscle

External oblique muscle (reflected)

FIG. 4.39

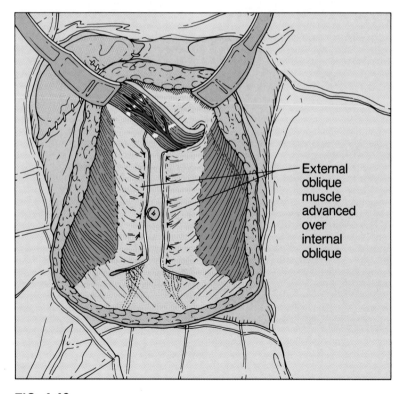

External oblique muscle advanced over internal oblique

FIG. 4.40

anterior rectus sheath, beginning at the costal margin and extending to the pubis *(Fig. 4.39)*. A second layer is then placed, advancing the external oblique muscle over the anterior rectus sheath and suturing them with three horizontal mattress sutures which are supplemented with running fine nylon. This maneuver is correct if the apparent bulging and flaccidity on the normal abdominal wall side is flattened and if it repositions the umbilicus close to the midline *(Fig. 4.40)*.

In bilateral reconstruction, the lateral fascia layers are sutured to the midline remnant as in the unilateral reconstruction, freeing the internal and external oblique layers separately.

With bilateral rectus flaps, it is important that both sides be closed simultaneously, placing one suture on the left and the next on the right side to prevent an overcorrection on one side that would make closure of the opposite side difficult or impossible.

If the repair is unusually tight, and if competent closure seems impossible to achieve, synthetic mesh (polypropylene or Marlex) has been used as an onlay graft to reinforce the abdominal closure. This can be placed from the costal margin down to the pubis or only in the infraumbilical region *(Fig. 4.41)*. We have not noticed any problems with this method of abdominal closure reinforcement.

Reconstruction of the Umbilicus

The new location for the umbilicus is determined on the abdomen and a "Y" or diamond incision is made there, extending the full thickness of the abdominal apron. A 5-cm diameter area around the "Y" or diamond is then defatted *(Fig. 4.42.A)*.

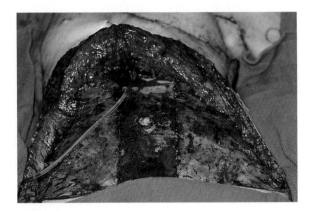

FIG. 4.41

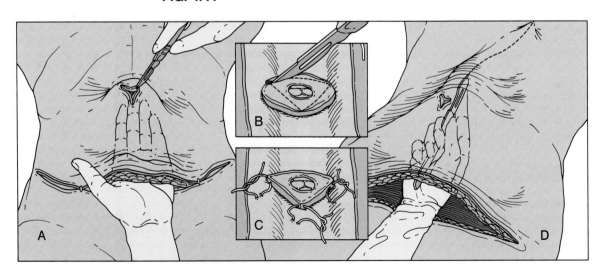

FIG. 4.42

The umbilical stalk is reattached to the anterior rectus sheath, again making every effort to place it in the midline *(Fig. 4.42.B)*. The umbilicus is narrowed appropriately and converted into a triangle, de-epithelializing the excess margins *(Fig. 4.42.C)*. The "V"-shaped skin from the "Y" abdominal incision is then sutured to the edges of the umbilicus with multiple interrupted sutures. This ensures a depressed umbilicus with a surrounding concavity which gives a normal and attractive appearance.

In addition, a midline depression is created in the upper abdominal flap from approximately the level of the xiphoid toward the umbilicus by cutting the fat with a knife almost down to the dermis. Additional defatting of the surrounding area can be accomplished with a suction-assisted lipectomy machine. The abdominal flap also is defatted in its lower border, particularly along the flanks, with the use of the suction lipectomy machine or by directly removing fat deep to Scarpa's layer.

The wound is then closed and suction catheters

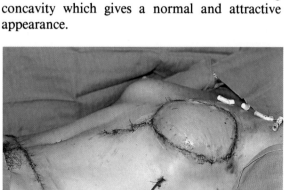

FIG. 4.43

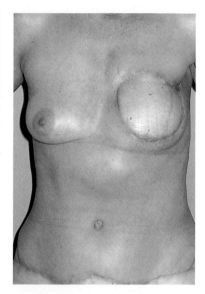

FIG. 4.44

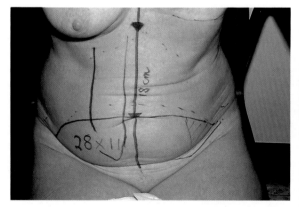

FIG. 4.45

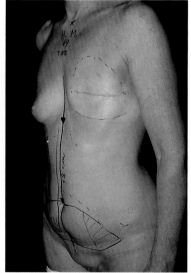

FIG. 4.46

are placed and brought out through the lateral edges of the incision *(Fig. 4.43). Figure 4.44* shows the postoperative view before nipple-areola reconstruction.

Clinical Cases

This technique is demonstrated in a 49-year-old woman, seen 1 year following a Patey-type mastectomy on the left side. She was thin, but had enough abdominal tissue to allow reconstruction of a breast of the same size as the other *(Figs. 4.45,* *4.46).* Due to excessive lordosis, her abdomen was rather prominent. Reconstruction was planned with a right flap.

The operation was performed according to Hartrampf, with a 3-cm strip of anterior fascia left on the muscle.[4] The lateral bands of the anterior fascia were detached from the muscle, which was totally taken as the pedicle of the abdominal flap *(Figs. 4.47, 4.48).* After transferring the flap, the muscle was replaced by Teflon mesh *(Figs. 4.49,* *4.50).* The flap was placed vertically and partly de-epithelialized to re-create the upper part of the

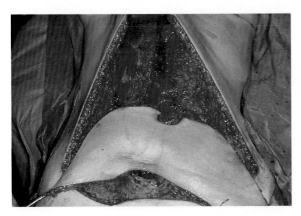

FIG. 4.47

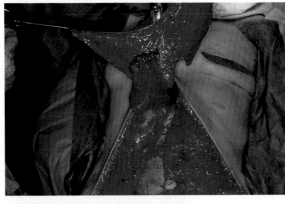

FIG. 4.48

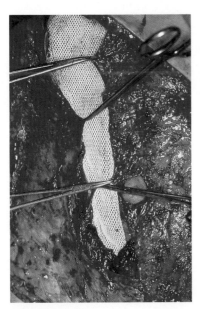

FIG. 4.49

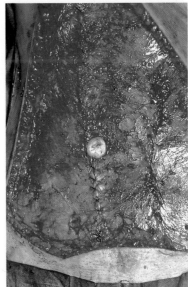

FIG. 4.50

breast *(Figs. 4.51, 4.52)*. Healing was uneventful.

Figure 4.53 shows the result after 2 months. The patient was able to sit without the help of the arms *(Fig. 4.54)*. Three months after the first operation, the areola and nipple were reconstructed with perineal skin, and two small implants were placed behind the breasts to slightly increase their volume. The result, 6 months later, is shown in *Figures 4.55, 4.56.*

The same principle was applied in a 53-year-old patient with a mastectomy on the right side *(Figs. 4.57, 4.58)*. She had a Pfannenstiel scar in the lower abdomen. The mastectomy scar was oblique and the skin relatively fibrous after irradiation. A left-side TRAM flap was used and, in this case, placed horizontally to give more width to the breast and to imitate the opposite one better *(Figs. 4.59, 4.60)*. Nearly 3 months later, the areola was

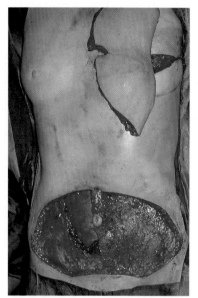

FIG. 4.51

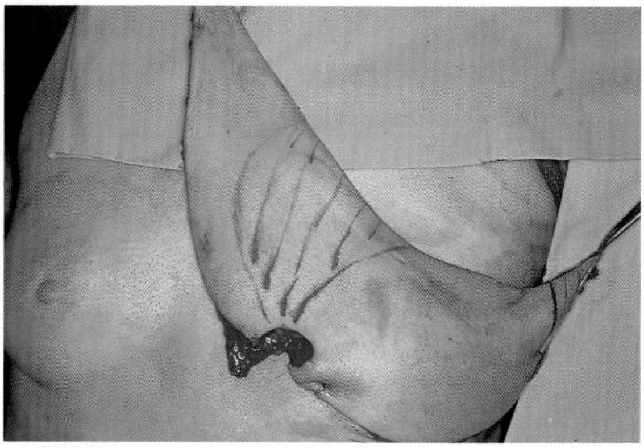

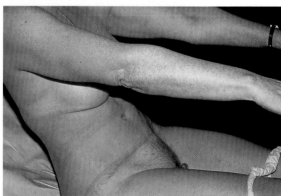

FIG. 4.52

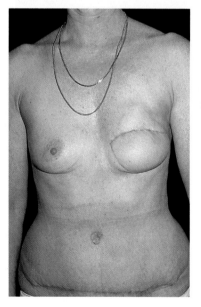

FIG. 4.53

FIG. 4.54

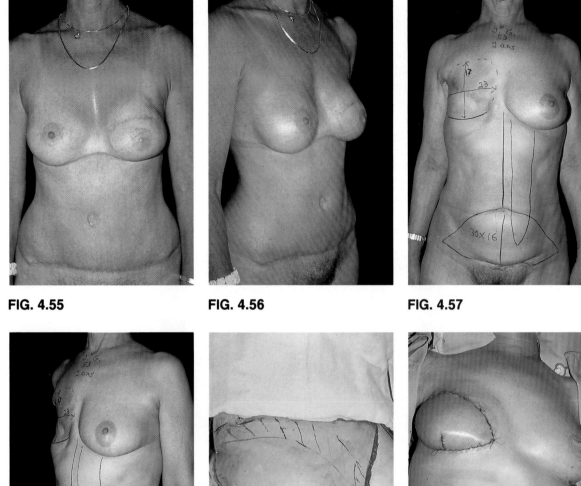

FIG. 4.55

FIG. 4.56

FIG. 4.57

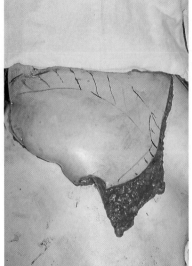

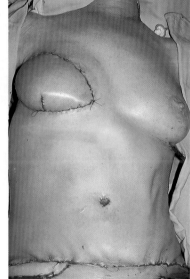

FIG. 4.58

FIG. 4.59

FIG. 4.60

reconstructed with perineal skin *(Fig. 4.61)*. The final result, 1 year after reconstruction, is shown in *Figures 4.62* and *4.63*.

Both cases had satisfactory results. In the first, the flap was placed vertically with the umbilical site medially. In the second case, the flap was placed horizontally with the umbilical site in the lower part of the chest wound, at approximately 6 o'clock, improving the shape of the breast by the wedge-shaped excision of skin.

This technique is recommended if more width is needed to make the breast, at least in women who do not have a major amount of excess abdominal skin. It should be stressed, however, that a flap with one pedicle is less safe when it is used horizontally, because some of the contralateral upper portion of the zone II flap is used to reconstruct the medial lower part of the breast. This has led to partial necrosis of that part of the flap in one of 11 cases. The flap was remolded after removal of the dead tissue on the second postoperative day. The result was satisfactory, but less projection of the breast was obtained. In cases when both sides of the abdomen must be used to produce a large and full breast, it is certainly safer to take a bilateral pedicle.

The decision of using one or two pedicles for the flap must be made considering different factors. A double pedicle makes the flap safer and permits the use of the whole abdominal tissue, but it

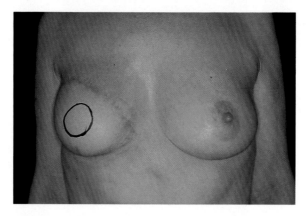

FIG. 4.61

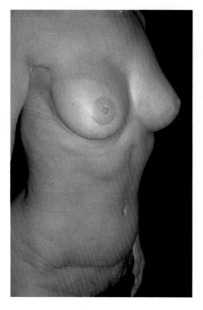

FIG. 4.62

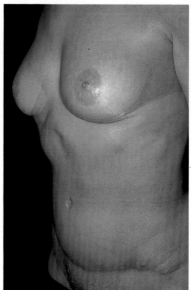

FIG. 4.63

increases the length of the operation, the amount of bleeding, and the risk of later abdominal complications. This should be especially taken into account in obese patients.

Although unilateral reconstructions with bilateral TRAM flaps are done more and more frequently, we are reluctant to perform them in obese patients with a relaxed abdominal wall. This is the best technique to create a full breast in patients who have little abdominal excess and also in those considered vascular high risks (smokers, patients with an irradiated sternal region, and older patients).

The following case demonstrates the advantages of the bilateral method. The patient had had a Halsted left mastectomy 9 years before presentation for a breast reconstruction *(Fig. 4.64)*. A simple implantation of a double lumen prosthesis containing 20 mg of prednisolone was first performed. Thinning of the skin and impending necrosis occurred after 4 months *(Fig. 4.65)* and a muscular latissimus flap was introduced under the pectoral skin while the implant was exchanged with another containing no cortisone. The result was satisfactory for several years but a capsular contracture developed progressively, as shown on a picture taken 4 years after the operation *(Fig. 4.66)*. The patient did not want any more surgery at that time, and the implant was extruded 4 years later *(Fig. 4.67)*.

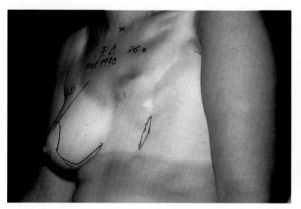

FIG. 4.64

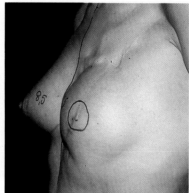

FIG. 4.65

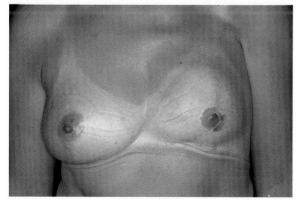

FIG. 4.66

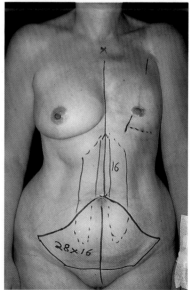

FIG. 4.67

The patient then agreed to have a bilateral TRAM flap, which used both muscles *(Fig. 4.68)*. A Teflon mesh placed on both sides was covered by suturing the remaining anterior fasciae *(Figs. 4.69, 4.70)*. The remnants of the rectus abdominis were very fibrous. This was confirmed on histologic sections *(Fig. 4.71)* which showed some muscular fibers dissociated by fat and fibrous tissue. A large abdominal flap adequately replaced the missing breast and pectoralis tissues. Two months after the operation, the patient could easily sit without the help of her hands *(Fig. 4.72)*. The result is shown 5 months after the repair and 2 months after nipple-areola reconstruction *(Figs. 4.73–4.75)*.

When dealing with failed previous reconstruc-

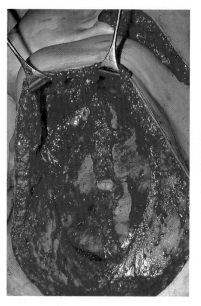

FIG. 4.68

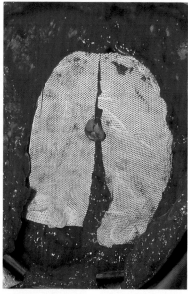

FIG. 4.69

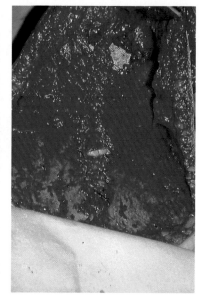

FIG. 4.70

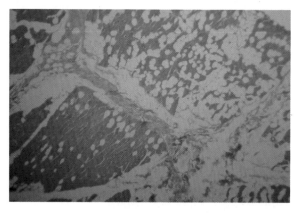

FIG. 4.71

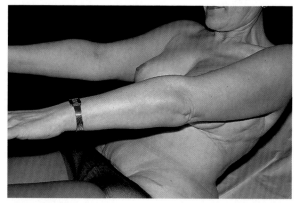

FIG. 4.72

tion, it is better to remove all the abnormal breast tissue and re-create a totally new breast. This avoids the patchwork aspect otherwise re-produced.

The patient shown in *Figures 4.76* and *4.77* had a latissimus flap procedure performed in another country several years earlier. The prosthesis was rejected. The result was poor and difficult to correct due to the high position of the latissimus flap and the x-ray damage of the medial part of the breast. The damaged skin was removed and the skin portion of the latissimus flap was de-epitheli-

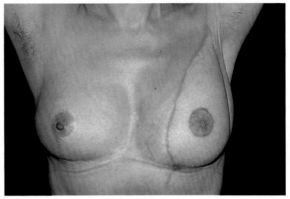

FIG. 4.74

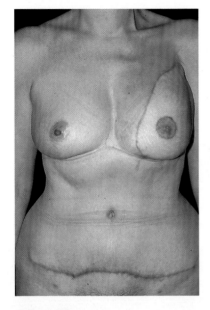

FIG. 4.73

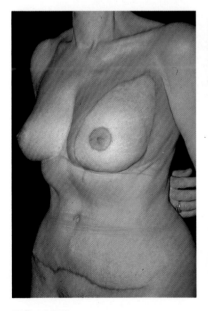

FIG. 4.75

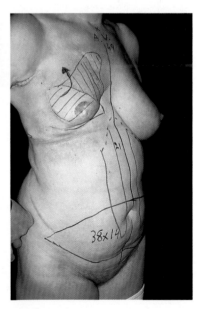

FIG. 4.76   FIG. 4.77

alized and pushed into the preaxillary defect *(Figs. 4.78, 4.79)*. A bilateral TRAM flap was prepared *(Fig. 4.80)* and used almost totally for the reconstruction of the whole breast *(Fig. 4.81)*. Five days after the operation, the patient was discharged with a satisfactory result *(Figs. 4.82–4.84)*.

Because the flaps have an unpredictable blood supply, the bilateral TRAM flaps are becoming increasingly popular. A good indication of a bilateral flap for unilateral reconstruction is the patient without known high risk of complication for whom a unilateral flap has been planned and in whom the superior epigastric artery is neither easily palpated nor demonstrated by Doppler during dissection of the pedicle. In such a case, a second pedicle can be added before the abdominal dissection is started, and the whole reconstruction may be saved by doubling the blood supply of the flap.

The bulk of the upper part of the pedicle(s) has been a matter of concern for our patients. It disappears in a few weeks by muscle atrophy if all the nerves, up to the eighth, have been cut during the operation. A secondary correction occurs as one re-creates the medial extension of the inframammary fold with the suction-assisted lipectomy and percutaneous sutures.

Variations Due to Abdominal Scars

Before the decision can be made to use rectus abdominis muscle flaps for breast reconstruction, the abdominal wall must be evaluated. Abdominal wall incisions may compromise the vascularity of a TRAM flap.

Vertical Lower Midline Scar

The rectus abdominis perforators usually are not disrupted in a vertical midline incision. These incisions, however, interrupt collateral flow across the midline. To permit a symmetrical excision when a transverse ellipse is elevated, the nonvascularized contralateral tissue is elevated in the ellipse and

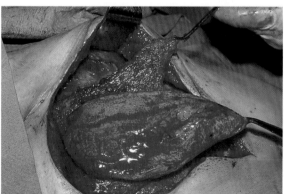

FIG. 4.78

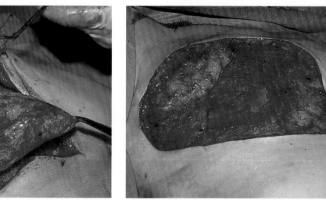

FIG. 4.79

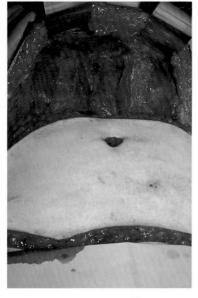

FIG. 4.80

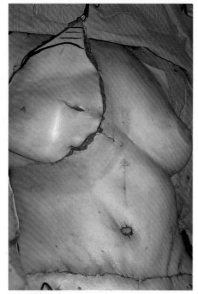

FIG. 4.81

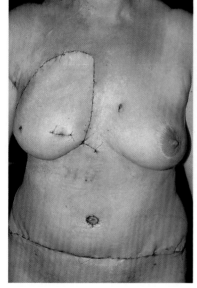

FIG. 4.82

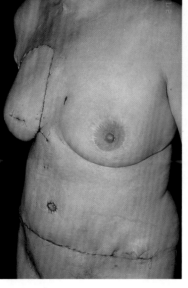

FIG. 4.83

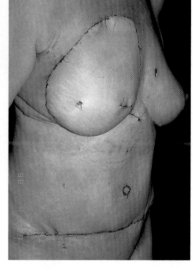

FIG. 4.84

discarded. We use a TRAM flap with a double pedicle when more than the ipsilateral tissue is needed.

Figures 4.85–4.87 show a 55-year-old woman who had a bilateral modified radical mastectomy for bilateral breast carcinoma. She underwent radiation and chemotherapy.

Figure 4.88 shows some convexity and excess skin of the abdomen. There is a well-healed lower midline scar, as well as bilateral hernia-type scars.

Bilateral reconstruction of the breast with a bilateral transverse island abdominal flap was indicated *(Fig. 4.89)*. The outline of the transabdominal flap was higher than usual because of the inguinal hernia incisions, which were oblique and extended above the anterior superior iliac spine. The superior line was located approximately 3 cm above the umbilicus, extended inferiorly below the anterior superior iliac spines, and included a portion of the inguinal incisions.

Flap bisection proceeded along the lower midline scar and extended above the umbilicus *(Fig. 4.90)*. The entire rectus muscle was elevated with each abdominal flap, as well as a 4-cm section of anterior rectus fascia extending from the pubis toward the costal margin *(Fig. 4.91)*. The TRAM flaps were passed on the ipsilateral side.

Figure 4.92 reveals the donor defect. *Figures 4.93* and *4.94* show the anterior rectus fascia. The reconstruction of the abdominal wall was identical

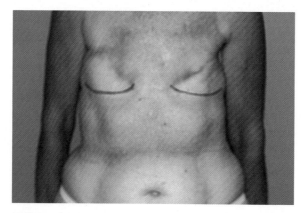

FIG. 4.85

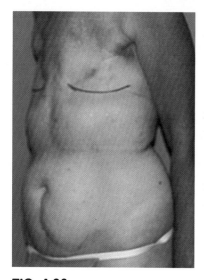

FIG. 4.86

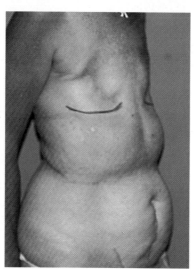

FIG. 4.87

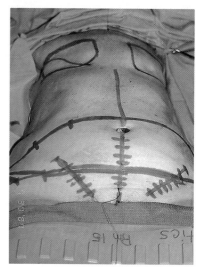

FIG. 4.88

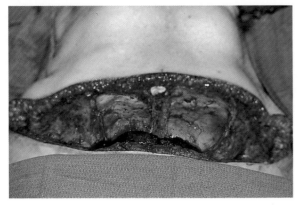

FIG. 4.89

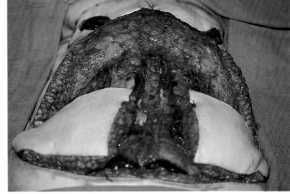

FIG. 4.90

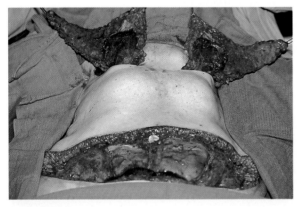

FIG. 4.91

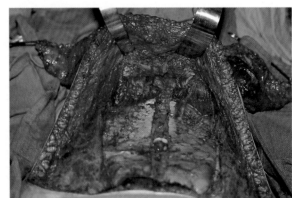

FIG. 4.92

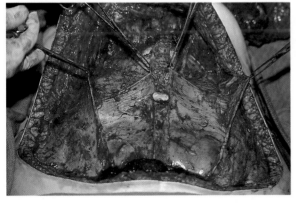

FIG. 4.93

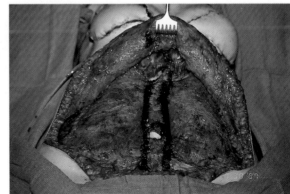

FIG. 4.94

to those described in the previous section. Secure closure of the abdominal wall was obtained, although use of Marlex mesh as a reinforcement was indicated. The mesh was placed from the xiphoid to the pubis *(Fig. 4.95)*. The immediate postoperative view appears in *Figure 4.96.*

Figures 4.97–4.99 show the nice result 10 months after bilateral reconstruction.

Paramedian Scar

A rectus abdominis flap is not considered reliable when it is located on the side of a prior paramedian incision. These incisions divide the midportion of the rectus abdominis muscle and often injure the rectus abdominis perforators. They denervate the rectus in the area medial to the incision, causing atrophy of the muscle. Tissue distal to scars should be discarded to ensure a healthy flap.

The appendectomy scars (right lower quadrant) vary greatly in length and location. The options include:

- Right breast reconstruction, use the TRAM flap with contralateral pedicle.
- Left breast reconstruction, use the TRAM flap with ipsilateral pedicle.
- Bilateral breast reconstruction, use the TRAM flap taken higher on the abdomen to get well-vascularized tissue.

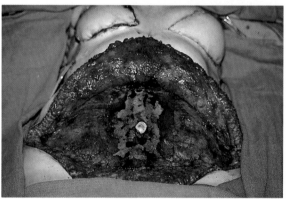

FIG. 4.95

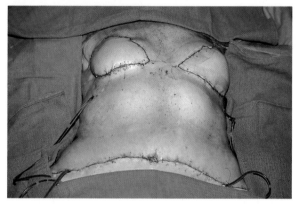

FIG. 4.96

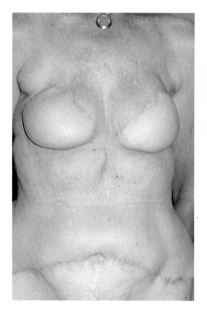

FIG. 4.97

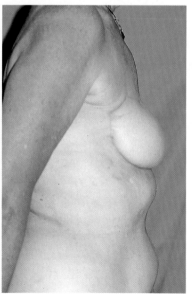

FIG. 4.98

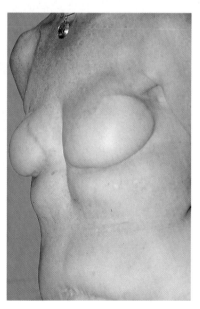

FIG. 4.99

Figures 4.100–4.102 show a 53-year-old woman who had a simple mastectomy 10 years earlier for carcinoma of the breast. She shows a well-healed mastectomy scar, a convex abdomen, and a lower paramedian right scar (appendectomy) which pre- vented using the contralateral flap. The contralateral side of the flap was excised, except for a small portion demarcated as a triangle at the level of the lower paramedian incision.

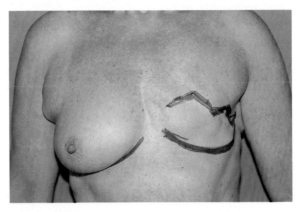

FIG. 4.100

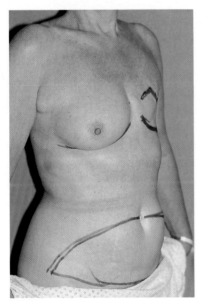

FIG. 4.101

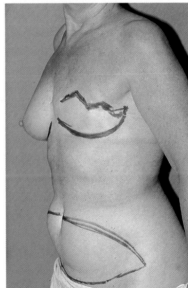

FIG. 4.102

Figures 4.103–4.105 show the patient 10 months after reconstruction of the left breast with an ipsilateral transverse island abdominal flap.

Transverse Abdominal Scar

These scars usually divide any underlying rectus abdominis muscle. A previous abdominoplasty divides the rectus abdominis perforators and contraindicates a TRAM flap, either upper or lower.

The Pfannenstiel approach for pelvic operations is preferable. This dissection usually divides the lower rectus abdominis perforators below the umbilicus. For patients who have a Pfannenstiel scar, a midabdominal or upper transverse rectus abdominis flap is safer.

A transverse or subcostal incision for cholecystectomy (Kocher's incision) usually divides the underlying rectus abdominis muscle and its epigastric system. Occasionally the incision extends a variable distance across the midline, and some of the opposite rectus abdominis muscle may be divided.

TRAM flap options with transverse subcostal scars include:

- Right breast reconstruction, use the TRAM flap with a contralateral vascular pedicle.
- Left breast reconstruction, use the TRAM flap with an ipsilateral vascular pedicle.
- Bilateral breast reconstruction, use free flap breast reconstruction on one side and a conventional TRAM flap on the other side.

The use of the upper bilateral TRAM flaps or a combination of one upper and one lower TRAM flap has the disadvantage of a midabdominal scar or a large "Z" scar on the abdomen and a shorter vascular pedicle which will require costal cartilage

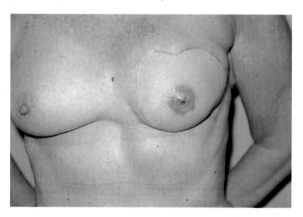

FIG. 4.103

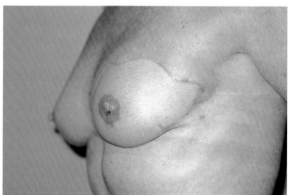

FIG. 4.104

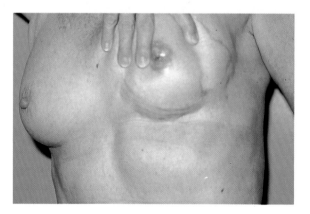

FIG. 4.105

removal. For the upper abdominal incisions that cross the midline and divide both rectus muscles, a double free flap for bilateral reconstruction may be a good option—when expert microvascular teams are available.

Figures 4.106 and *4.107* illustrate the case of a 62-year-old woman who underwent a modified radical mastectomy for right breast carcinoma. The patient had a small, slightly ptotic left breast, and the abdomen showed a right subcostal incision (cholecystectomy), lower midline incision (hysterectomy), and appendectomy scar.

Figures 4.108 and *4.109* show the right breast reconstruction with a contralateral hemi-TRAM flap. Sufficient tissue was available to permit reconstruction.

BILATERAL TRAM FLAP BREAST RECONSTRUCTION

The TRAM flap operation is an excellent alternative for reconstruction of the bilateral mastectomy defect. The abdominal wall flaps are appealing to many patients because they reduce excess abdominal wall tissue while providing a source of skin and soft tissue for breast reconstruction.

In addition, this technique has certain advantages over other procedures: the tissue for both breasts is taken from one abdominal wound, the operation is performed without turning or repositioning the patient from a supine position, and two surgeons can work simultaneously and thereby reduce operative time.

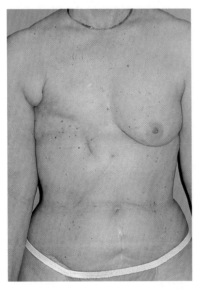

FIG. 4.106

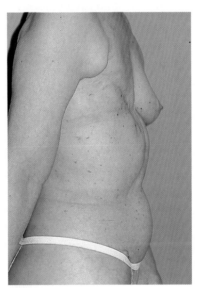

FIG. 4.107

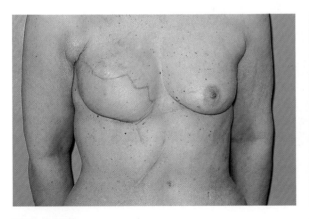

FIG. 4.108

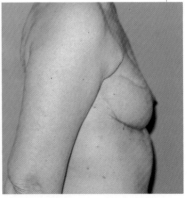

FIG. 4.109

Use of the TRAM flap procedure is limited in the small, thin, nulliparous patients. They usually do not have excess abdominal wall tissue available to rebuild two adequate breasts without the use of silicone prostheses.

Preoperative Planning

The patient was a 46-year-old woman who had had a modified radical mastectomy on the right breast for intraductal carcinoma, and a prophylactic subcutaneous mastectomy on the left side 7 months later.

Chest

During preparation for bilateral reconstruction, if the mastectomy scars are not at approximately the same level or if they are oriented in dissimilar directions, it is best to ignore one or both scars and to design new incision lines that are similar.

Markings are made for each breast to define the proper breast pockets and to determine the amount of tissue required *(Figs. 4.110, 4.111)*. In the case illustrated, more tissue is needed on the right (the side of the modified radical mastectomy) to make the new breasts the same size.

Abdomen

The lower abdominal ellipse is marked as in the unilateral reconstruction, and is the same as that described previously. The superior limits of the flap are drawn just above the umbilicus, and the inferior limits above the suprapubic crease. These limits are extended to meet symmetrically and lateral to the anterior superior iliac spine on both sides.

Surgical Technique

Chest

The mastectomy scar on the right side is excised. The contralateral mastectomy is performed at the same operative session as the breast reconstruction, with the incision designed to match the mastectomy scar on the right side. The chest skin flaps are elevated to the limits of the mastectomy. The inframammary adhesion is not disturbed on either side.

A tunnel is dissected from the medial breast pocket on both sides into the lower sternal area. The tunnel joins a common channel through the epigastrium connecting with the lower abdominal incision.

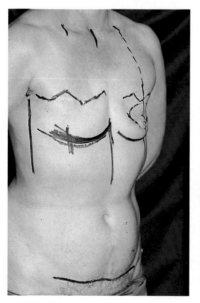

FIG. 4.110

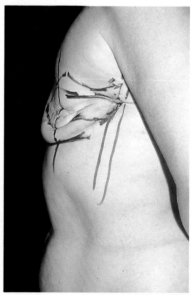

FIG. 4.111

Abdomen

The abdominal flaps are elevated in the same manner as in the unilateral reconstruction, except that the vascular pedicle is preserved on both sides and the transverse abdominal island flap is split in the midline *(Figs. 4.112, 4.113)*.

With a bilateral reconstruction, it is even more important to save the medial and lateral fascial segments to allow a secure primary abdominal wall closure *(Fig. 4.114)*.

After both sides of the abdominal flap are elevated, both flaps are passed through the common epigastric tunnel *(Fig. 4.115)*. To facilitate closure, the lateral fascial layers are closed to the midline fascia in alternating fashion, as described previously.

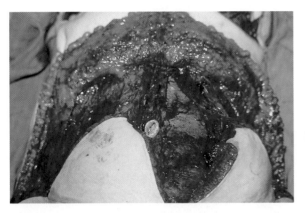

FIG. 4.112

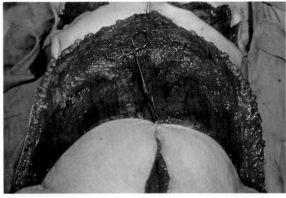

FIG. 4.113

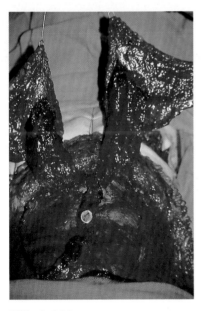

FIG. 4.114

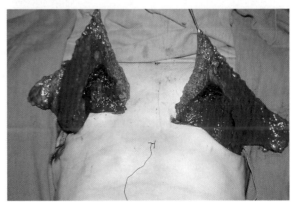

FIG. 4.115

Figure 4.116 shows the internal oblique muscle closed. The dissection of the external oblique muscle is seen in *Figure 4.117*. *Figure 4.118* shows that the external oblique muscle and the rectus sheath have been repaired in two layers.

Shaping the Breast

The abdominal flaps are secured to the upper limits of the mastectomy pocket as described in the unilateral reconstruction. In the bilateral reconstruction, less tissue is available for each side for obtaining size and projection.

During the bilateral reconstruction, it is important to set the upper attachment of the flap and the inframammary crease at the same level on both sides and to try to achieve equal size in the two breasts *(Fig. 4.119)*.

Figures 4.120–4.122 show the same patient with nipple-areola reconstruction 1 year following bilateral reconstruction.

After elevating the bilateral flaps, one may either cross the pedicles or maintain them ipsilaterally. Crossing the pedicles and flaps is attractive, but we discourage it because the added bulk of one muscle may compromise the venous return of the other flap. This has happened to us on two occasions; fortunately, we noticed it intraoperatively and immediately resorted to ipsilateral passage.

With ipsilateral use of the flaps, these must be rotated at least 270° to make the skin side appear

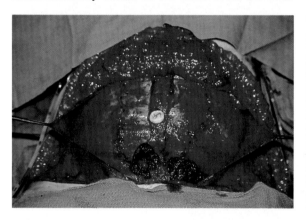

FIG. 4.116

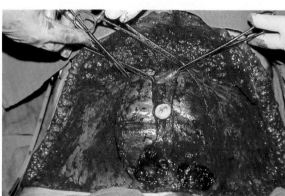

FIG. 4.117

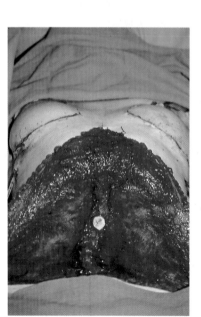

FIG. 4.118

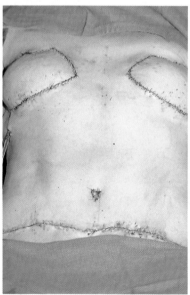

FIG. 4.119

BREAST RECONSTRUCTION WITH FLAPS

externally. Such a twist can be accomplished safely. The rotation can be clockwise or counterclockwise, but one should avoid at all costs a double fold of the muscle (see Chapter 14).

For molding the breast, the umbilical site is placed at 4, 5, or 6 o'clock. The flap is transversely oriented and an attempt is made to give projection to the mound.

BILATERAL TRAM FLAP RECONSTRUCTION—MASTECTOMY OF THE CONTRALATERAL BREAST AT RISK

The factors that confer high-risk status to the contralateral breast in a patient who undergoes mastectomy, as determined by the American Cancer Society,[1] are listed in *Table 4.1.*

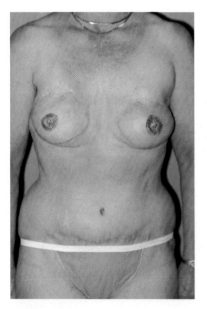

FIG. 4.120

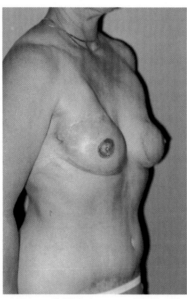

FIG. 4.121

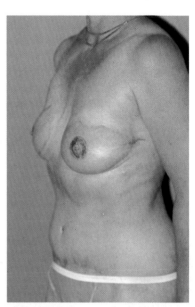

FIG. 4.122

Table 4.1
Patients at High Risk for Cancer of the Contralateral Breast

Positive family history in a first-order relative (sister, maternal aunt, mother, grandmother), particularly if cancer developed premenopausally or is bilateral.

Certain types of cancer in the primary breast (e.g., lobular carcinoma), which increase the risk to the opposite breast.

Multifocal disease.

Biopsy of the opposite breast showing lobular or ductal hyperplasia with atypia.

Early menarche and late menopause.

Nulliparity.

Birth of first child at 30 years of age or older.

Mammograms of the dense Wolfe classification type, making interpretation of changes difficult.[8]

The patient at high risk for a second breast cancer is managed either by constant close observation or by prophylactic mastectomy. Close collaboration and discussion between the oncologic surgeon, the plastic surgeon, the patient, and the patient's family are required. The final decision, however, must be one that is most consistent with the patient's feelings.

The goals for management of the contralateral breast in postmastectomy reconstruction are (1) to prevent or to detect as early as possible a subsequent carcinoma, especially in the woman considered to be at high risk for subsequent carcinoma, and (2) to provide symmetry with the reconstructed breast contour. The advantage of a bilat-eral reconstruction is that the tissue which could be used for a unilateral reconstruction may be divided and used for both breasts.

Clinical Case

The patient in *Figures 4.123* and *4.124* is a 38-year-old woman with a strong family history of breast cancer who had a modified radical mastectomy on the right side for carcinoma. The left breast is quite large, ptotic, and difficult to examine. A simple left mastectomy was performed and a bilateral TRAM flap was planned.

Figures 4.125–4.127 show the patient 6 months after breast reconstruction with bilateral TRAM

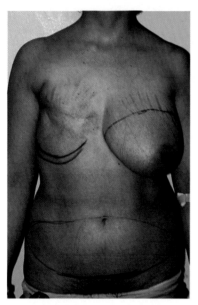

FIG. 4.123

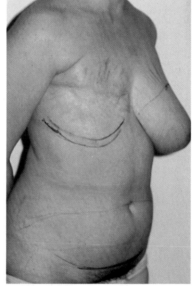

FIG. 4.124

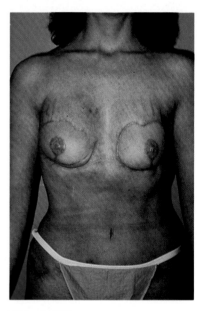

FIG. 4.125

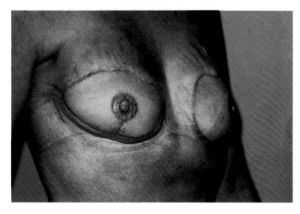

FIG. 4.126

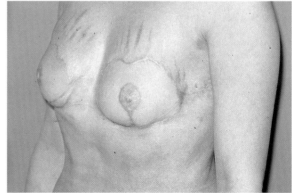

FIG. 4.127

BREAST RECONSTRUCTION WITH FLAPS

flaps. The surgical procedure and abdomen wall closure were identical to those described in the previous section.

Ipsilateral flaps were used. The left mastectomy was performed by way of an incision similar to that on the right side; a considerable amount of superfluous skin was discarded.

REFERENCES

1. Bostwick J III: *Aesthetic and Reconstructive Breast Surgery.* St. Louis, CV Mosby, 1983.
2. Carramenha e Costa M, Carriquiry C, Vasconez LO, et al: An anatomic study of the venous drainage of the transverse rectus abdominis musculocutaneous flap. *Plast Reconstr Surg 1987;72:208.*
3. Duchateau J, Declety A, Lejour M: Innervation of the rectus abdominis muscle: implications for rectus flaps. *Plast Reconstr Surg 1988; 82(2):223.*
4. Hartrampf C: Abdominal wall competence in transverse abdominal island flap operations. *Ann Plast Surg 1984;12:139.*
5. Hartrampf C: *Transverse Abdominal Island Flap Technique for Breast Reconstruction After Mastectomy.* Baltimore, University Park Press, 1984.
6. Leis H Jr, Raciti A: The search for women at high risk, in Stoll B (ed): *Risk Factors in Breast Cancer, Volume 2.* Chicago, Year Book, 1976, 207.
7. Scheflan M, Dinner MI: The transverse abdominal island flap. Part I. Indications, contraindications, results, and complications. *Ann Plast Surg 1983;10:24.*
8. Wolfe JN: Breast patterns as an index of risk for developing breast cancer. *Am J Roentgenol 1976;126:1130.*

CHAPTER·5

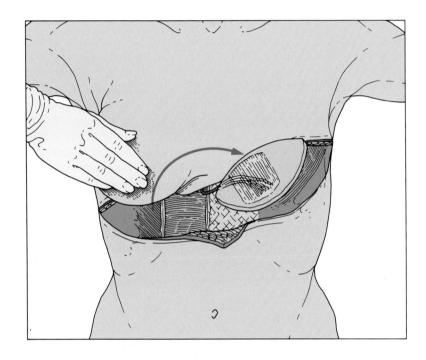

Contralateral Upper Rectus Flap for Breast Reconstruction

The contralateral upper rectus flap for breast reconstruction was introduced at approximately the same time as the transverse island abdominal flap.

Indications

The objective of the procedure is to use tissue from the contralateral normal inframammary area, where there is excess skin of the same color and texture. The flap is transposed to the mastectomy side by rotating it 180°. A portion of the upper rectus muscle with the superior epigastric vessel should be included.

Advantages

This procedure is useful in young women who have had no children and who have a relatively flat lower abdomen. The technique has been applied for selected patients with unilateral burn scar contractures and also for those with postradiation lumpectomy defects, particularly on the medial aspect of the breast.

Disadvantages

The procedure has certain drawbacks, which include the technical difficulty of elevating the flap and transposing it 180°. If the reconstruction requires a large mound or placement of the skin island high on the chest, it is necessary to free the internal mammary artery for a considerable distance in a subperichondrial fashion underneath the costal margin. In almost every case the silicone implant has to be inserted during the reconstruction procedure.

Surgical Technique

Figure 5.1 shows the island flap in the normal submammary fold and the clockwise rotation required to reach the oblique mastectomy scar. The scar is reopened and a pocket reaching to the submammary fold is created.

Although not indicated in the diagram, it is best if the ellipse is truncated at the midline of the abdomen to gain better access to the anterior rectus sheath as well as the rectus muscle. The flap is outlined laterally to the anterior axillary line. Elevation is begun at that point to the level of the anterior rectus sheath. The lower abdominal flap is dissected on top of the rectus fascia, which is divided transversely to the midline to expose the rectus muscle. The muscle and the fascia are tran-

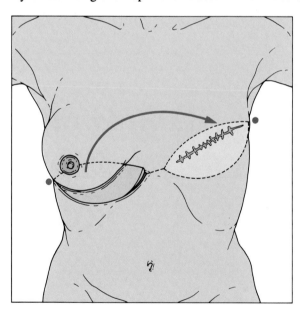

Fig. 5.1 *Reproduced from Gant TD and Vasconez LO[1] with permission of the publisher.*

sected approximately 2 cm below the lower edge of the skin flap, which is freed to the costal margin from the midline and from its lateral attachments. The entire flap is circumscribed, and the origin of the rectus muscle is divided from the costal margin. Thus, the flap with a portion of the muscle is converted into an island *(Fig. 5.2)*.

At this point the flap cannot be transposed to the contralateral side because of the very short vascular pedicle of the superior epigastric vessel. Now begins the most difficult part of the dissection. The internal mammary artery and its continuation as the superficial epigastric system shows a variable entrance into the rectus muscle. This entrance is not next to the xiphoid, but more likely about 3 to 4 cm laterally to it. One may localize the artery and vein by using a Doppler unit. On rare occasions it can be seen or felt.

It is essential to free the internal mammary artery for a considerable distance under the superichondrium to allow the flap to be transposed. We recommend removing the seventh costal cartilage, as well as additional cartilages as necessary, after they are freed in a subperichondrial fashion. When

necessary to achieve additional length for movement of the flap, the perichondrium has to be carefully incised as far laterally as possible. Each time it will be necessary to check that the axillary tip of the flap transposes and reaches as far laterally as the contralateral anterior axillary line.

Unless accomplished earlier, the mastectomy scar is opened. A subcutaneous dissection is performed to the inframammary fold. In almost every case, a silicone implant of appropriate size to match the opposite breast is inserted at this time. A tension-free closure is performed.

Monitoring of the blood supply to the flap is essential at all times, particularly after insertion of the silicone implant. The implant may put excessive traction on the vascular pedicle, which will make the flap blanch and require further dissection underneath the costal margin.

Once the flap has been adequately transposed by opening the skin across the midsternum and the appropriate silicone implant has been inserted, closure is performed without drains. It is preferable to sacrifice a certain amount of skin so that the flap is positioned at the inframammary fold.

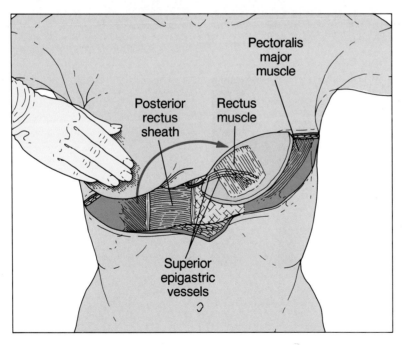

Fig. 5.2 *Reproduced from Gant TD and Vasconez LO[1] with permission of the publisher.*

Closure of the secondary defect is then performed by advancing the rectus sheath with the muscle and reattaching it to the costal margin whenever possible. Doing so avoids a relative emptiness in the upper abdomen.

Incisions across the sternum have not presented problems such as hypertrophy or excessive redness.

Figures 5.3 and *5.4* show a young woman with a right mastectomy whose breast was reconstructed with a contralateral upper rectus abdominal flap *(Figs. 5.5, 5.6).* The skin island was placed exactly at the inframammary fold and the second-ary scar is nicely hidden in the submammary fold. The scar across the sternum has not hypertrophied.

REFERENCES

1. Gant TD, Vasconez LO: *Postmastectomy Reconstruction,* p.165. Baltimore, Williams & Wilkins, 1980.
2. Vasconez LO, Psillakis J, Johnson-Giebeik R: Breast reconstruction with contralateral rectus abdominis myocutaneous flap. *Plast Reconstr Surg* 1983; 71:668.

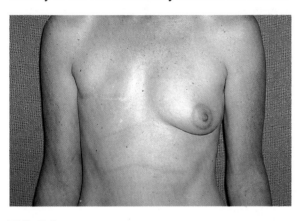

FIG. 5.3

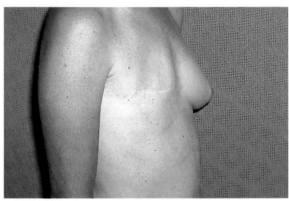

FIG. 5.4

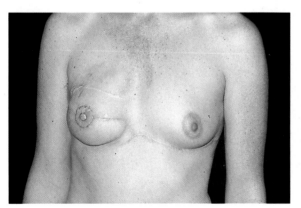

FIG. 5.5

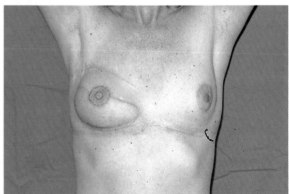

FIG. 5.6

CHAPTER · 6

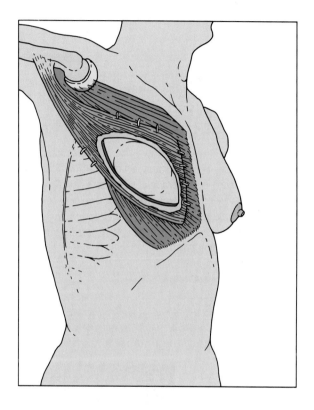

Immediate Postmastectomy Breast Reconstruction

Indications

Virtually any patient can be considered a candidate for immediate breast reconstruction based solely on the stage of her disease. Immediate reconstruction may be extremely important for the psychologic well-being of the woman in a more advanced disease stage, than for a woman with stage I disease whose surgery may well have been curative.

The psychologic benefits of immediate reconstruction lessen the emotional morbidity of the mastectomy wound. In some patients any delay in reconstruction may aggravate their anxiety and depression, and complicate the emotional symptoms of mastectomy.

Advantages

Immediate reconstruction offers the mastectomy patient a single-stage procedure and does not affect or interfere with a postoperative adjuvant therapy schedule. Wound healing has not been a problem. The implant or autogenous tissue reconstruction is incorporated into the body image more readily at this point in recovery.

Disadvantages

The operating time is prolonged by immediate reconstruction depending upon the technique undertaken. The use of autogenous tissue techniques may add 4 to 6 hours to the time required for the mastectomy. In addition, blood transfusion is usually necessary in the autogenous tissue technique.

Morbidity of immediate reconstruction is increased if the mastectomy flaps are thin and an implant is placed submuscularly or even subcutaneously below the flaps. Another insult to an already compromised flap is the greater potential for ischemic necrosis. In the TRAM operation, the most sophisticated of breast reconstructions, delayed wound healing or partial loss of the flap, fat necrosis, or total loss of the breast reconstruction may occur.

Some patients will seem disappointed when comparing the reconstructed breast with the normal breast. These patients have not had the opportunity to see the mastectomy deformity and are less appreciative of the reconstructed breast.

Intraoperative Management

Immediate postmastectomy reconstruction is best performed by a team. The oncologic surgeon takes full responsibility for the extent of the mastectomy and the choice of incisions. The reconstructive team usually waits until the breast has been removed.

The team approach to TRAM flap elevation and breast molding has proved to be efficient and effective. Two surgeons work to elevate the TRAM flap for transposition while a third surgeon prepares the axillary wound and flap inset site. In im-

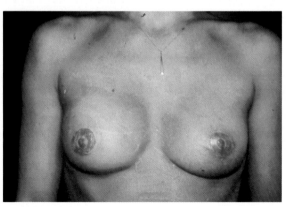

FIG. 6.1

mediate reconstruction, it is important to close the empty space of the axillary dissection by approximating the latissimus dorsi muscle to the chest wall and suturing the subcutaneous tissue of the lateral skin flap to the mid- and anterior axillary line. The evaluation of the viability of the mastectomy skin flaps is important. The edges of these flaps are debrided in all cases to avoid the chance of necrosis or delayed healing.

Methods

The methods for immediate breast reconstruction include implants and/or expanders, autogenous tissue reconstruction, and autogenous tissue plus a permanent implant.

Implants and Expanders

The use of implants for breast reconstruction can be subdivided into three categories: immediate submuscular implants, tissue expansion with subsequent permanent implants, and the permanent expander prosthesis.

Immediate submuscular implants are placed through the mastectomy wound much as one would do an augmentation mammaplasty. *Figure 6.1* shows submuscular implants 5 years postop.

Tissue expansion with subsequent permanent implants as the selected technique for immediate reconstruction involves an effort to match the reconstructed breast to the large intact breast.

The third type of implant reconstruction involves the use of the permanent expander prosthesis. This procedure involves an expander with a valve apparatus which can be removed under local anesthesia once the desired breast volume has been reached. *Figures 6.2* and *6.3* show a patient 8 months after immediate breast reconstruction with Becker-type permanent expander implants.

Autogenous Tissue Reconstruction

This option provides the closest approximation in character, color, and texture of the tissue it replaces. The procedure is free from the potential of capsular contracture because no prosthesis is needed. The abdominoplasty necessary to close the donor site is viewed as a bonus for most patients.

The disadvantage of the TRAM flap procedure is that it is a technically difficult operation. Potential herniation at the donor site and an insensible breast mound are also potential problems. The surgical procedures are the same as those described in previous sections.

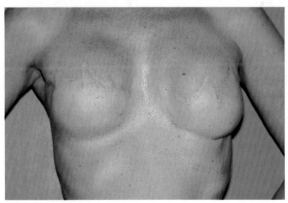

FIG. 6.3

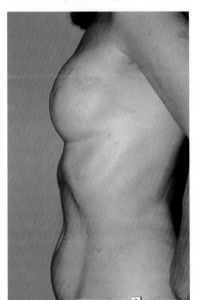

FIG. 6.2

Figures 6.4–6.6 show a 45-year-old woman with infiltrating ductal carcinoma of the left breast, stage T$_2$ NoMo, who had a left modified radical mastectomy. *Figures 6.7* and *6.8* show the patient 5 months after immediate breast reconstruction with a lower transverse rectus abdominis flap.

Although it adds additional difficulty to immediate breast reconstruction, the TRAM flap may be transferred as a free flap or the gluteus maximus muscle and overlying cutaneous island may be harvested for the reconstruction. The free TRAM offers more convenience for positioning the patient to harvest the flap. Both the free TRAM and free gluteus maximus muscle reconstructions suffer, however, from positioning difficulties when the microvascular anastomosis in the axilla is performed.

The free TRAM provides two benefits over the standard muscle pedicled flap. There is no costal or epigastric bulge, and there is less donor site morbidity because only a small segment of rectus muscle is needed.

The benefits, however, must be weighed seriously against the potential disaster of an unrecognized anastomotic failure and loss of the entire TRAM.

Autogenous Tissue plus a Permanent Implant
Although this technique brings additional autogenous tissue into the mastectomy wound for reconstruction, the implant provides the breast mound.

Figures 6.9 and *6.10* show a patient 5 months after latissimus dorsi myocutaneous flap reconstruction.

This technique is not frequently used today for two reasons. First, the experience and general acceptance of tissue expansion has obviated the need for latissimus dorsi muscle coverage at the time of immediate reconstruction. Second, the concept of total autogenous reconstruction with the TRAM flap has further reduced this choice as a reconstructive option.

Complications

Complications associated with implants include infection, extrusion or deflation of the implant, rupture or migration of the implant, and inability to achieve symmetry.

Skin slough of the mastectomy flaps may occur with or without exposure of the prosthesis. Capsular contracture complications associated with autogenous tissue reconstruction and the TRAM flap include partial to full skin slough or necrosis of the flap, wound infection with delayed healing, fat necrosis, and abdominal wall hernia.

Conclusion

Satisfactory techniques are available for immediate reconstruction depending upon the patient's wishes and the judgment of the surgeon. We be-

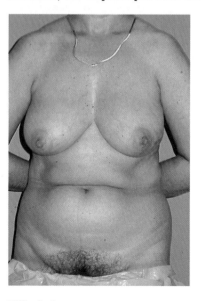

FIG. 6.4

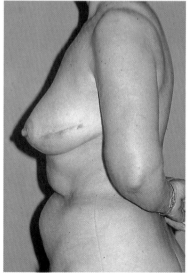

FIG. 6.5

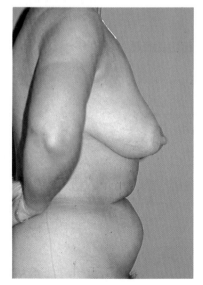

FIG. 6.6

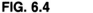

lieve there is no contraindication for immediate breast reconstruction if the patient is a candidate for ablative surgery. Our personal preference in immediate reconstruction is autogenous tissue reconstruction with the TRAM flap. This bias grew from experience in the aesthetic improvement and the overall quality of the reconstruction compared with the significant contracture rate associated with prosthetic implants, and has not diminished over the years.

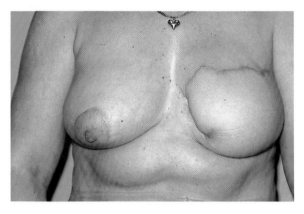

FIG. 6.7

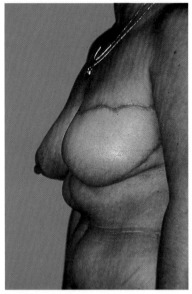

FIG. 6.8

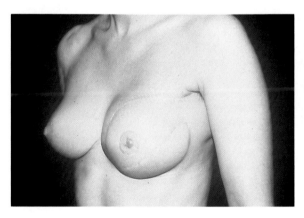

FIG. 6.9

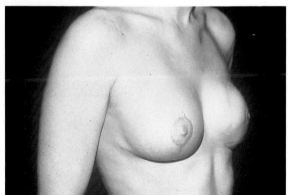

FIG. 6.10

CHAPTER·7

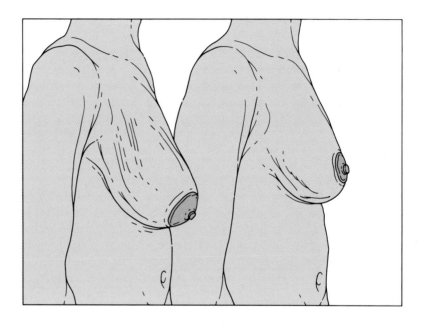

Procedures on the
Opposite Breast

PREOPERATIVE DECISIONS

When the opposite breast is considered after unilateral mastectomy for cancer, the three concerns that surgeons face are oncologic risk, adjustment of the volume and shape of the reconstructed breast to obtain symmetry, and possible sharing of the nipple-areola complex when fashioning the areola of the reconstructed side.

Oncologic Risk

Before any reconstruction begins, the oncologic risks have to be evaluated. Some surgeons advise prophylactic subcutaneous mastectomies with prosthetic replacements for all patients. Among those with unilateral mastectomies, the overall risk of developing carcinoma in the opposite breast is approximately 15% (compared with 7% risk in the normal Caucasion population). Such a rate is too low for us to perform prophylactic subcutaneous mastectomies in all cases, because these operations often yield disappointing results. Simple mastectomies are preferable for high-risk cases, such as lobular carcinoma in the amputated breast, extensive fibrocystic disease, and history of breast cancer in the family.

Opposite Breast Adjustment

In cases other than those stated earlier, and if the preoperative mammography is normal, the opposite breast is adjusted to the reconstructed breast when necessary. In this regard, our operations have included mastopexy (37%), reduction (22%), augmentation (12%), subcutaneous mastectomy (4%), reconstruction (3%), mastectomy (3%), and no surgery required (19%).

In the case of simple and latissimus reconstructions in which the amputated breast is reconstructed with an implant, the opposite breast is always adjusted during the same operation. Symmetry in volume can be judged at this time. In TRAM flap reconstruction, the opposite breast is corrected during the second-stage operation only because, in these cases, symmetry with the reconstructed side is easier to evaluate several weeks after surgery.

In all patients, the volume of the breasts is decided according to the general proportions of the patient rather than by the volume of the opposite breast, which often is too large. This is why, in implant reconstructions, the side to be reconstructed is operated on first during the initial stage, unless the opposite side requires only a correction of shape.

The usual techniques of mammaplasty are slightly modified to reduce the forward projection of the breast and to preserve the whole areola, if a later sharing is intended. A moderate volume of the breast is recommended to prevent, as much as possible, future ptosis of the mammary gland which can spoil the symmetry achieved with the reconstructed breast.

Nipple-Areola Complex Sharing

If large enough, the nipple-areola complex will be the donor site for the reconstructed side. The areola is shared about 3 months after reshaping the

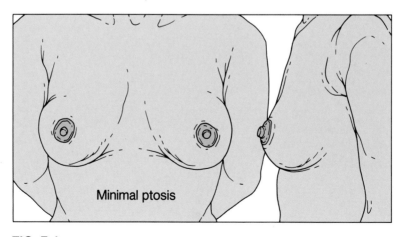

FIG. 7.1

breast. The outer surface is taken as a free graft, and the donor breast is reshaped by an inferior V excision.

MASTOPEXY

Mastopexy, or surgical correction of ptosis, involves elevation of the nipple-areola complex and tightening of the skin envelope to support the breast at a higher position. Symmetrical and naturally proportioned and positioned breasts are the goals of mastopexy.

Surgical Technique

Mastopexy incisions are longer than incisions for augmentation mammaplasty. They should be placed in the shadows on the lower side of the breast.

The surgical treatment of this condition involves a range of possible corrections based primarily on the nipple-areolar position and size, amount of excess skin, and breast volume. Mas-

topexy can also be combined with other techniques, such as breast augmentation or resection and reduction of breast parenchyma.

Correction of Breast Ptosis

The correction of ptosis is approached according to the classification or grade of the condition:

MINIMAL PTOSIS. The nipple-areola is above the inframammary crease, most of the gland is below nipple level, and there is a mild decrease in skin elasticity *(Fig. 7.1)*. In the mastopexy approach to corrections of minimal ptosis, one may use skin excisions and reshaping of the breast, repositioning of the nipple-areola, and later additional correction through the original scars if recurrence of the ptosis develops. Periareolar skin excision gives minimal skin tightening in patients with large areolae *(Fig. 7.2)*.

GRADE I PTOSIS. The nipple-areola is at the inframammary crease level, the gland position is behind the nipple-areola, and there is moderate

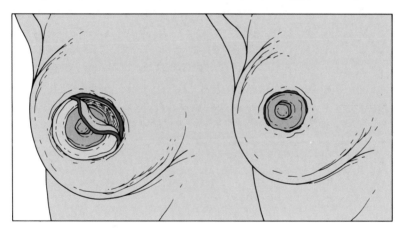

FIG. 7.2

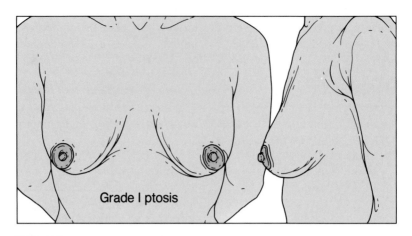

Grade I ptosis

FIG. 7.3

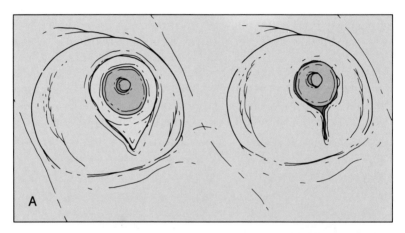

A

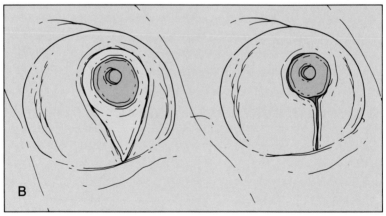

B

FIG. 7.4

decrease in skin elasticity *(Fig. 7.3)*. The mastopexy approach for correction of grade I ptosis includes periareolar skin excision with a short *(Fig. 7.4.A)* or long *(Fig. 7.4.B)* vertical ellipse which permits skin tightening and nipple elevation, but without an inframammary incision. *Figure 7.5* shows a patient with a grade I ptotic left breast and mastectomized right breast. She underwent breast reconstruction with an implant and ptosis reduction by way of a long vertical ellipse *(Fig. 7.6)*.

GRADE II PTOSIS. The nipple-areola is 1 to 3 cm below the inframammary crease, the gland is positioned behind the nipple-areola, and there is poor skin elasticity *(Fig. 7.7)*. *Figure 7.8* illustrates

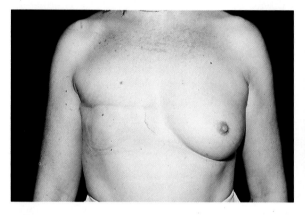

FIG. 7.5

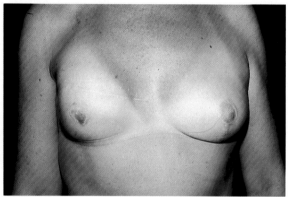

FIG. 7.6

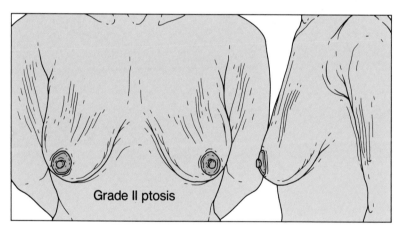

Grade II ptosis

FIG. 7.7

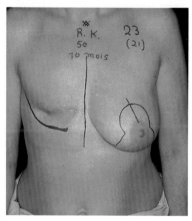

FIG. 7.8

the method used for correction of grade II ptosis, an approach with a vertical ellipse and a short horizontal ellipse. This tightens the breast and shortens the inframammary distance, while keeping the inframammary scar short *(Figs. 7.9, 7.10)*.

GRADE III PTOSIS. The nipple-areola is more than 3 cm below the inframammary crease and points downward, the gland is low and above the nipple-areola, and the skin is inelastic and stretched, with striae *(Figs. 7.11–7.13)*. The mastopexy approach to correction of grade III ptosis includes a vertical and horizontal excision designed to achieve maximal correction. The inframammary scar is longer *(Figs. 7.14–7.16)*.

Complications

Complications of mastopexy may include inadequate correction, recurrent ptosis, and asymmetries.

BREAST REDUCTION AND MASTOPEXY

Many of our patients underwent breast reduction by way of a modified Strömbeck technique[7] in which only the medial pedicle of the areola was used.

Another technique, developed more recently, not only reduces the length of the submammary scar, but is also safer and permits adjustment of the shape of the breast to the reconstructed side.

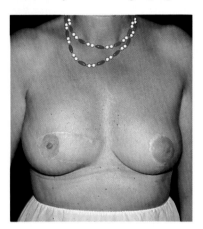

FIG. 7.9

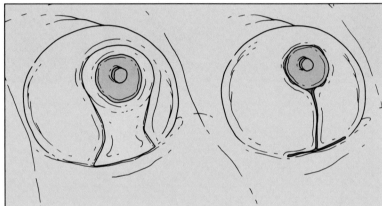

FIG. 7.10

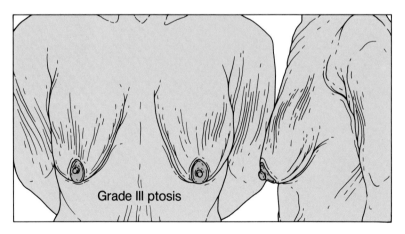

Grade III ptosis

FIG. 7.11

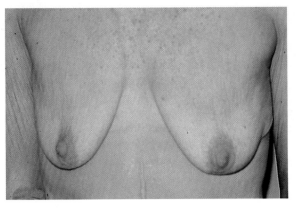

FIG. 7.12

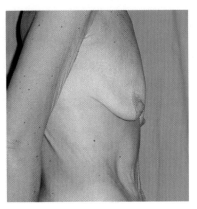

FIG. 7.13

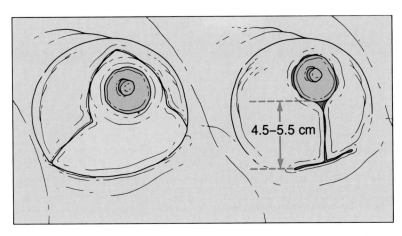

4.5–5.5 cm

FIG. 7.14

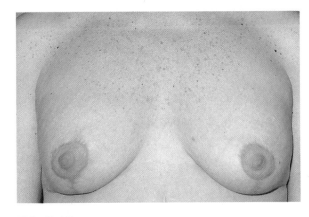

FIG. 7.15

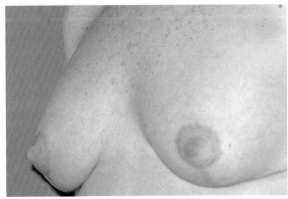

FIG. 7.16

This technique is based on the vertical mammaplasty proposed by Arie[1] and later improved by Lassus[5] and Marchac and Olarte.[6]

Preoperative Decisions

To obtain good symmetry, a drawing is performed before the operation on the standing patient. The submammary fold is located, and the new site of the nipple determined accordingly. The upper pole of the future areola is placed 2 cm above the new site of the nipple *(Fig. 7.17.A)*. The inner border of the future areola is located 8 to 12 cm from the midline, according to the size of the patient *(Fig. 7.17.B)*. The vertical axis of the breast is drawn under the submammary fold and a 4- to 6-cm horizontal line is placed 3 to 5 cm above it *(Fig. 7.17.C)*. By marking the natural midline of the breast, one can then pull it and mark the resection line in a plane even with the natural midline. Then

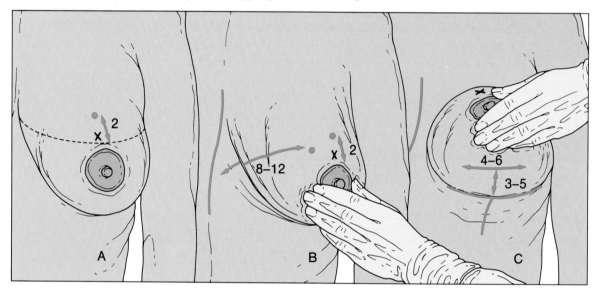

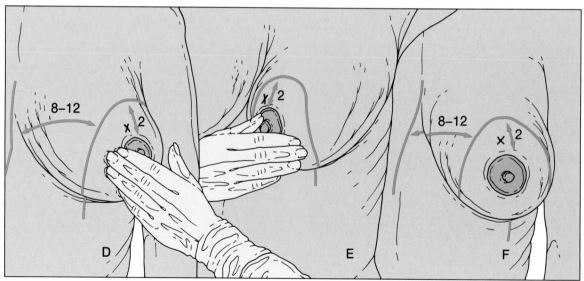

FIG. 7.17

the same is done for the opposite side of the breast *(Fig. 7.17.D,E)*. The portion that needs to be resected is shown in *Fig. 7.17.F*.

The area of skin limited by the drawing will be de-epithelialized in the upper part and removed in the lower part. By pinching the breast, one can appreciate the quantity of glandular tissue to be removed *(Figs. 7.18, 7.19)*. When the breast is pinched high, more tissue will be removed, there will be less tension around the areola, and the submammary scar will be longer. When the breast is pinched low *(Fig. 7.19)*, more tissue will be left in place, the tension on the areola will be greater, and the submammary scar will be shorter. Too much tension around the areola results in scar stretching. It is better to have a longer submammary scar that remains quite inconspicuous, as long as it does not pass beyond the new submammary fold.

Surgical Technique

The upper part of the area limited by the drawn circle *(Fig. 7.20)* is de-epithelialized up to 3 cm lower than the areola *(Fig. 7.21)*. The skin is incised laterally and the glandular tissue cut perpendicularly to the skin as far as the pectoralis fascia, leaving a wide upper dermoglandular pedicle for the areola. The breast tissue limited by the lat-

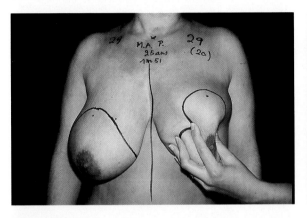

FIG. 7.18

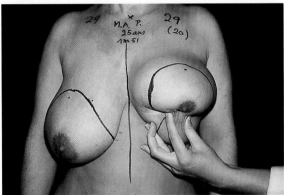

FIG. 7.19

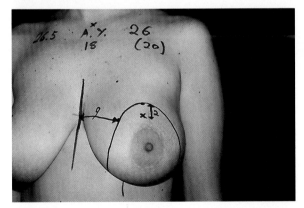

FIG. 7.20

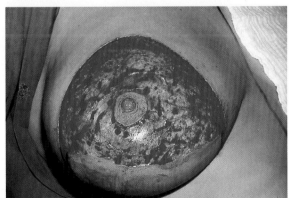

FIG. 7.21

eral incisions is detached from the lower part of the skin down to the submammary fold *(Fig. 7.22)*. The breast is then completely detached from the muscular plane to its upper pole *(Fig. 7.23)*. The excess tissue is excised from the lower part *(Fig. 7.24)* and, if necessary, from the superior part of the breast flap, at least 2 cm behind the areola *(Fig. 7.25)*. No glandular tissue is removed in mastopexy.

The remaining areolar flap is lifted and sutured to the muscular fascia at the upper pole of the breast, creating a temporary high bulge and reduc-

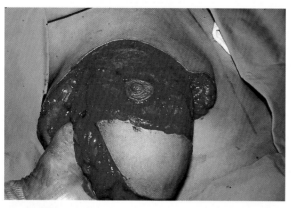

FIG. 7.22

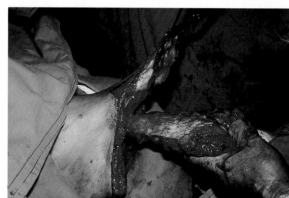

FIG. 7.23

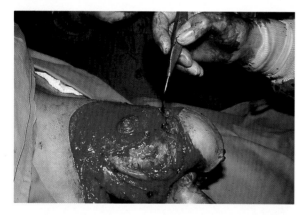

FIG. 7.24

FIG. 7.25

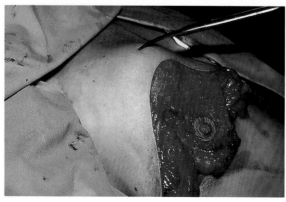

FIG. 7.26

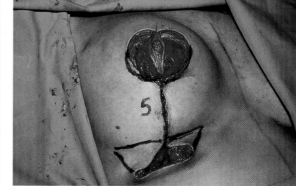

FIG. 7.27

ing tension on the lower part of the breast *(Fig. 7.26)*. The lateral pillars of the breast are approximated under the areola with absorbable sutures *(Fig. 7.27)*. The lower part of the gland is anchored to the thoracic fascia. This is essential to prevent the breast from sliding behind the submammary fold.

After trimming the adjacent skin, running absorbable and nylon sutures are placed around the areola to obtain a regular circle. The submammary fold is placed 5 to 7 cm under the areola along the lower pole of the breast by drawing a line 3 to 12 cm long according to the size of the lower dog-ear *(Fig. 7.28)*. The excess skin and fat is excised along the new submammary fold *(Fig. 7.29)*. The resulting submammary scar is not visible outside the breast after reduction *(Fig. 7.30)*.

If the breast is reduced to match a breast reconstructed with an implant only (which often is flatter than ideal), it is advisable to create a breast with less projection by increasing the size of the arch

around the areola. This method gives a variety of possibilities for adjusting the opposite breast with reconstruction procedures.

BREAST AUGMENTATION AND MASTOPEXY

When there is some ptosis after glandular involution, a combination of prosthetic implantation and mastopexy is indicated. If the ptosis is not severe, the glandular tissue is left intact and the skin is only reshaped. As usual, the implant is placed behind the muscle before closing the submammary suture. These cases often give a satisfactory symmetry with the side reconstructed with an implant.

REDUCTION MAMMAPLASTY

The goal of reduction mammaplasty is to reduce, recontour, and reshape the breasts. With this oper-

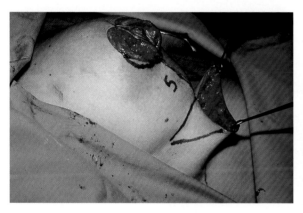

FIG. 7.28

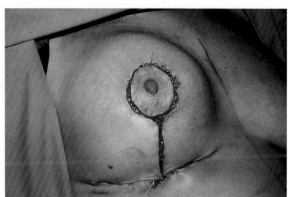

FIG. 7.29

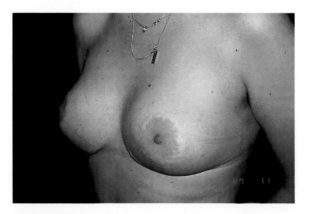

FIG. 7.30

ation the breasts are made smaller, the nipple-areola is repositioned upward, and the excess skin is removed *(Fig. 7.31)*. The expected results from this operation are attractiveness and symmetry.

Macromastia of Large Breasts

The symptoms indicated in reduction mammaplasty include mastodynia, shoulder grooving, pressure symptoms on the brachial plexus, pain in the cervical and upper thoracic spine, intertriginous eczema around the inframammary fold, and psychosocial problems.

Indications for this procedure are giant virginal hypertrophy *(Fig. 7.32)* after pregnancy when the breasts do not involute to their previous volume, and after menopause if the patient has large breasts with significant ptosis. In a mastectomy patient with large breasts, symmetry can be obtained by reducing the size of the opposite breast.

Preoperative Decisions

A careful history, physical examination, and laboratory tests are made before the operation. Prospective mammography is recommended for patients older than 35 years and for all patients who have had a mastectomy for breast cancer.

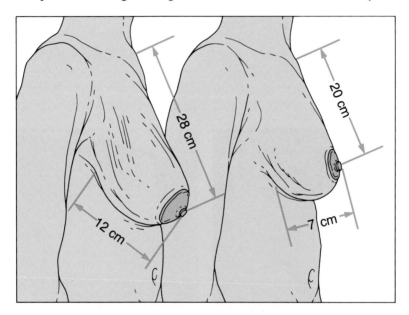

FIG. 7.31

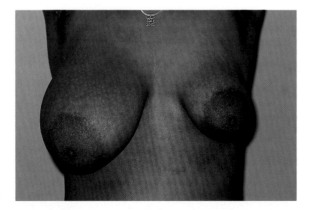

FIG. 7.32

Surgical Technique

Superior Pedicle Technique

This technique is used for breasts with modest to moderate hypertrophy requiring reductions of 200 to 1,000 g. The nipple-areola repositioning should be 8 cm or less from its previous site *(Fig. 7.33.A)*. Breast tissue resected from the lower pole repre-sents a major reduction with this technique *(Fig. 7.33.B)*. A vertical cut and lateral resection of the deep portion effectively narrow the breast when the inverted-T incision is closed *(Figs. 7.33.C)*. Although the deep lateral resection divides some central musculocutaneous perforators, vascularity to the remaining breast is preserved medially, lat-erally, and superiorly *(Fig. 7.34)*.

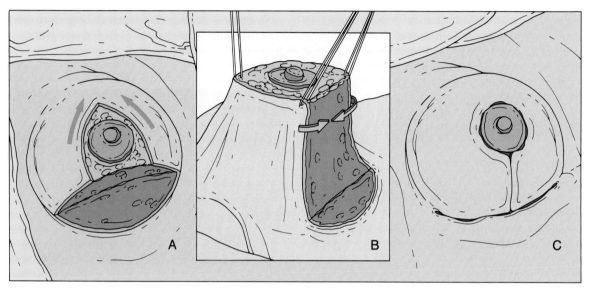

FIG. 7.33

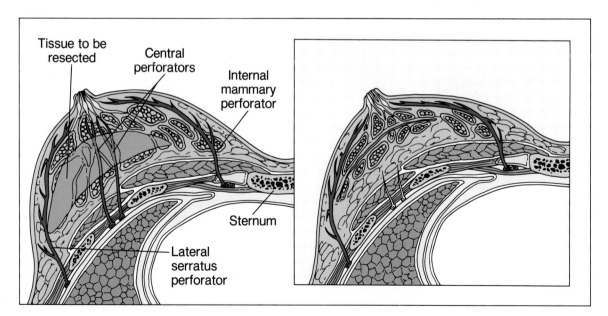

FIG. 7.34

Inferior Pedicle Technique

When the breasts are wide, pendulous, or large, and require reductions of 600 to 2,000 g, the inferior pedicle technique is useful. The key to this technique is preservation of a central breast mound *(Fig. 7.35)* containing the nipple-areola on a volume of central breast tissue primarily nourished by central perforating intercostal arteries *(Fig. 7.36)*. Medial, lateral, and direct muscular arteries also supply this central breast tissue. An inferior dermal pedicle that extends to the fascia pectoralis is preserved. The breast tissue is resected medially, laterally, superiorly, and inferiorly around the central breast mound *(Fig. 7.37.A)*. This is a more complex operation than the superior pedicle technique because the resections are performed in several areas. The free segment of the pedicle is then sutured to the fascia pectoralis. The skin envelope is advanced medially and inferiorly over the pedicle coning the breast *(Fig. 7.37.B)*. This maneuver minimizes the medial and lateral extension of the transverse incision. The new nipple-areola site is then determined over a dermal base, 4 cm above the inframammary line *(Fig. 7.37.C)*.

Complications

The complications of reduction mammaplasty are infections, hematoma, nipple-areolar loss *(Fig. 7.38)*, scars, nipple malposition, asymmetry, and inadequate breast reduction.

Clinical Case

Figures 7.39 and *7.40*: views before we implanted a 270-cc prosthesis and reduced the opposite side, and 2 months later, before capsulotomy and nipple-areola reconstruction with the other nipple-areola.

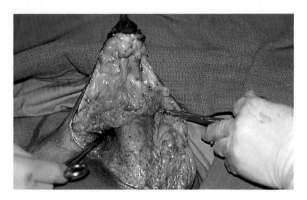

FIG. 7.35

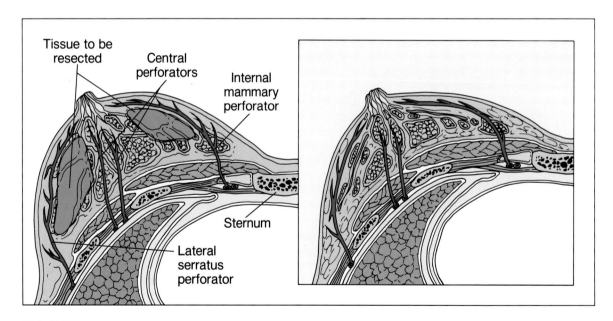

FIG. 7.36

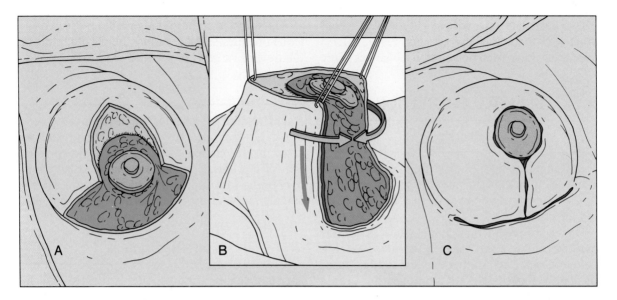

FIG. 7.37

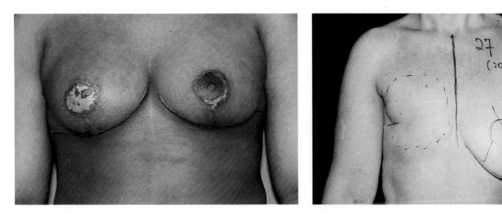

FIG. 7.38

FIG. 7.39

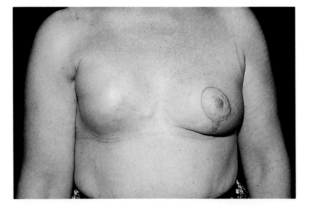

FIG. 7.40

Two years later, the patient's areola was reconstructed as a columellar graft *(Fig. 7.41)*. After 3 years, there have been no additional changes *(Figs. 7.42, 7.43)*.

BREAST AUGMENTATION

History

Breast augmentation using a free dermafat graft from the buttocks began about 1945 in the United States.[3] The results were impaired by resorption and infection.

The use of prosthetic material, such as Ivalon® and Etheron® sponges, began in the late 1950s. Silicone bags appeared during the next decade (those filled with silicone gel were introduced by Cronin and Gerow[4] in 1963). With various useful modifications they remain the implants now in use. In 1970 Ashley[2] introduced polyurethane-covered silicone prostheses, either empty, filled with saline at the time of surgery, or prefilled with silicone gel.

Indications

Augmentation is indicated when the breast size is not in aesthetic proportion with the body. These cases include patients who have a major involution of the breasts after pregnancy and lactation, hypoplasia and minimal breast development, or augmentation of the small normal breast to match a postmastectomy reconstruction with an implant.

Contraindications

Any undiagnosed lump should be treated first. In patients with more severe ptosis of the breast, a mastopexy is to be performed either first or simul-

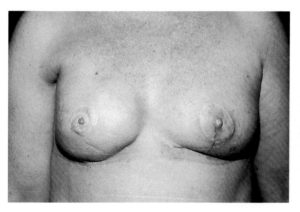

FIG. 7.41

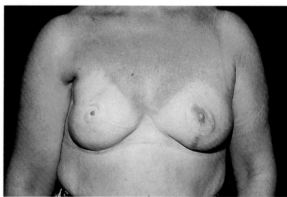

FIG. 7.42

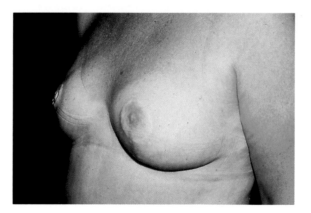

FIG. 7.43

taneously. The lower age limit for breast augmentation is 18; there is no older limit.

Implants

Soft silicone gel bags of various shapes and sizes can be used *(Fig. 7.44),* either nonprefilled, half-filled, or prefilled, and in regular profile, oval, or elongated.

Surgical Technique

General anesthesia or local infiltration plus sedation is used. After scrubbing and draping, the location of the submammary fold is marked, as well as the midline and the extension of the submusculofascial dissection *(Fig. 7.45).* We use a partially submuscular augmentation of the breast by inserting the implant behind the pectoralis major mus-

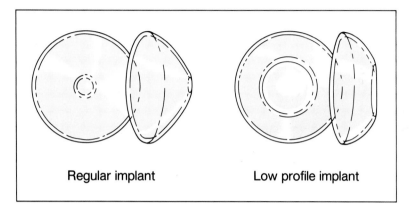

Regular implant   Low profile implant

FIG. 7.44

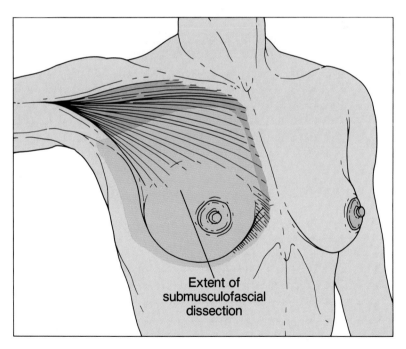

Extent of
submusculofascial
dissection

FIG. 7.45

cle, which covers the upper three quarters of the implant only *(Fig. 7.46)*. The implant is introduced by squeezing it into the pocket. Suturing is accomplished in layers, using separate stitches on the fascia but not including the pectoralis. The skin is approximated by a subcuticular running suture.

In postoperative management, use of a brassiere is not recommended in the first 1 to 2 postoperative weeks because it can elevate the implant to an unacceptable level. After 3 to 4 days the patient is encouraged to massage the implant toward the desired shape and position.

The incisions often used for breast augmentation are inframammary, periareolar, axillary, and abdominal *(Fig. 7.47)*.

Inframammary Incision

The inframammary approach leaves a well-located scar in a natural fold. The incision is 3.5 to 4 cm long *(Fig. 7.48)*. It allows direct access to the retromammary area and the musculofascial layer, thus enabling the creation of a precise pocket for implants of any size. Hemostasis is easier to achieve and the scar is controllable.

In the submusculofascial technique, the prosthe-

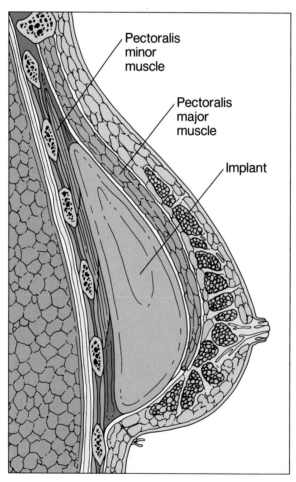

Pectoralis minor muscle

Pectoralis major muscle

Implant

FIG. 7.46

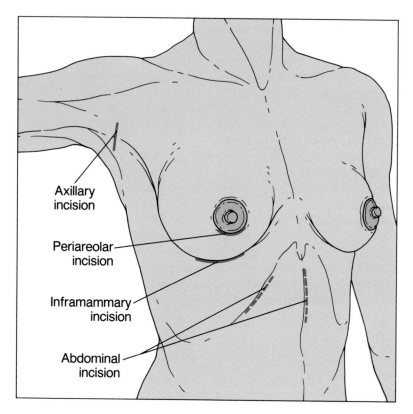

Axillary
incision

Periareolar
incision

Inframammary
incision

Abdominal
incision

FIG. 7.47

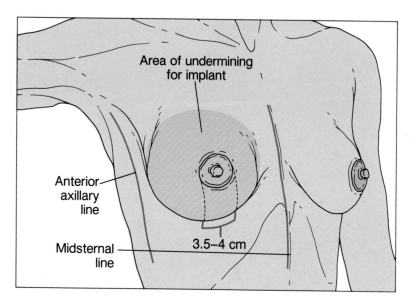

Area of undermining
for implant

Anterior
axillary
line

Midsternal
line

3.5–4 cm

FIG. 7.48

sis is placed beneath the pectoralis major muscle *(Fig. 7.49)*. In the subglandular technique, the undermining is done entirely above the pectoralis major and serratus muscles, and below the breast tissue itself. It is an easy plane to dissect, usually avascular *(Fig. 7.50)*.

The percentage of capsular contracture in augmentation mammaplasty is about 15%. In a subcutaneous mastectomy, the rate of capsular contraction is over 50%. Placement of the implant under the pectoralis muscle is thought to lessen the incidence of capsular contracture.

Unfavorable results of augmentation may include occasional adhesion of the pocket to the upper part of the muscle and lifting of the implant with contraction of the pectoralis. Pressure from the implant can cause atrophy or compression of the breast tissue. Implant slipping below the submammary fold also happens occasionally. Extrusion of the implant is rare.

Periareolar Incision

A semicircular incision 3.5 to 4 cm long is made at the inferior margin of the areola. The fat and gland are then incised down to the pectoralis

major muscle. Either a submuscular *(Fig. 7.51)* or subglandular *(Fig. 7.52)* pocket is dissected. Hemostasis may sometimes be difficult to achieve. The scar may be excellent, but if it becomes hypertrophic it is much more visible than an inframammary scar.

Axillary Incision

The incision for such a procedure is 4 to 6 cm long in the hairbearing midaxillary area and should follow the direction of the normal crease lines *(Fig. 7.53)*. Sharp dissection to the subcutaneous tissue is continued until the edge of the pectoralis major muscle is identified; the dissection continues either above or below the muscle. The introduction of the implant might be more difficult. This is a good approach when only a small augmentation is required. The scars are usually fine and easily concealed. Higher infection rates have been reported with this approach.

Abdominal Approach

When performing any aesthetic procedure on the abdomen, such as abdominoplasty or scar revision of the upper quadrants, an opportunity is provided

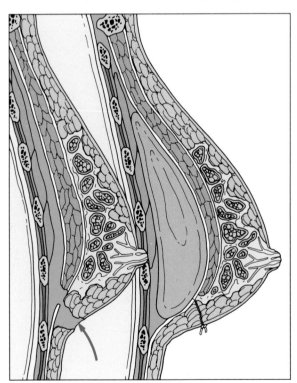

FIG. 7.49

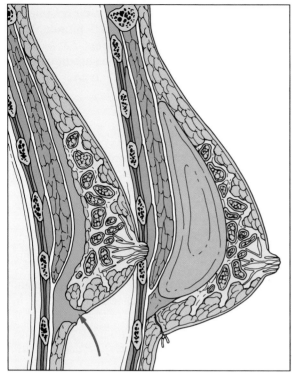

FIG. 7.50

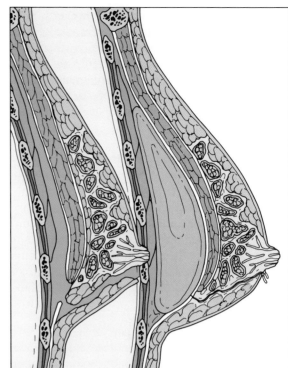

FIG. 7.51

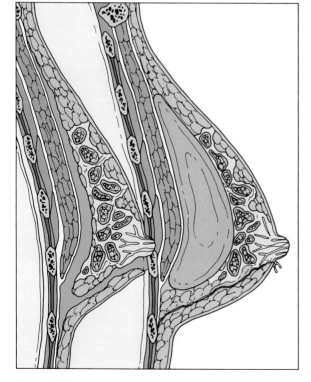

FIG. 7.52

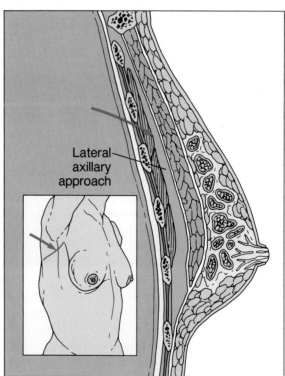

Lateral axillary approach

FIG. 7.53

for possible insertion of mammary implants. Subpectoral undermining is the easiest way to create the pocket for the prosthesis. One or two stitches are very important to prevent slipping of the implants, especially when they are small. We do not recommend the abdominal approach except in special circumstances, because it is such an involved procedure.

Complications

Complications of breast augmentation include operative bleeding, hematoma, infection, fibrotic capsular formation, sensory changes, temporary anesthesia in the nipple-areola complex, and hypersensitivity of the nipple. Scars and keloids are rare. Occasionally, an unaesthetic result occurs because of incorrect implant size and incorrect positioning. Fortunately, all these complications are infrequent.

Clinical Case

Figure 7.54 shows the patient before simple implantation of a 250-cc prosthesis and augmentation of the other side. Five months later, the patient presented with a strong capsular contraction and upper displacement of the implant *(Fig. 7.55)*. A drawing of the skin to be de-epithelialized to form the new submammary fold was performed

(Fig. 7.56). The patient is shown after completion of the operation *(Fig. 7.57)* and 5 months later, before areola reconstruction *(Fig. 7.58)*. Seven months later, the patient had a recurrent capsular contraction which pushed the breast up *(Fig. 7.59)*.

REFERENCES

1. Arie G: Una nueva técnica de mastoplastia. *Rev Latinoam Cirug Plast 1957;3:23.*
2. Ashley FL: A new type of breast prosthesis. *Plast Reconstr Surg 1970;45(5):421.*
3. Bames HO: Augmentation mammaplasty by lipo-transplant. *Plast Reconstr Surg 1953; 11:404.*
4. Cronin TD, Gerow FJ: Augmentation mammaplasty: a new "natural feel" prosthesis. *Int Congr Ser 1963;66(1):41.*
5. Lassus C: Reduction mammaplasty with short inframammary scars (letter). *Plast Reconstr Surg 1986;77(4):680.*
6. Marchac D, Olarte G de: Reduction mammaplasty and correction of ptosis with a short inframammary scar. *Plast Reconstr Surg 1982;69(1):45.*
7. Strömbeck JO: Reduction mammaplasty. *Surg Clin North Am 1971;51(2):453.*

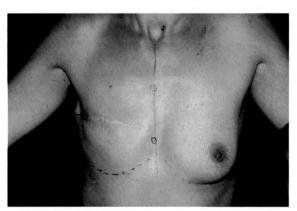

FIG. 7.54

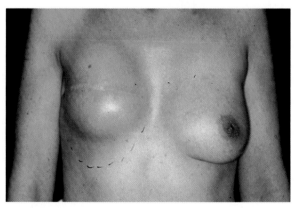

FIG. 7.55

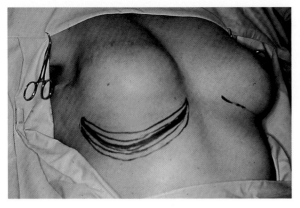

FIG. 7.56

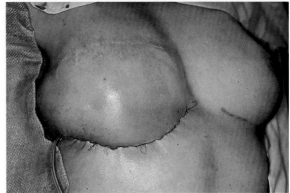

FIG. 7.57

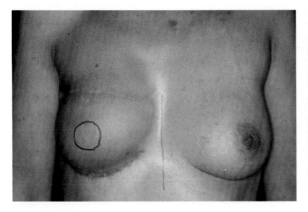

FIG. 7.58

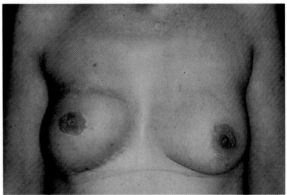

FIG. 7.59

CHAPTER·8

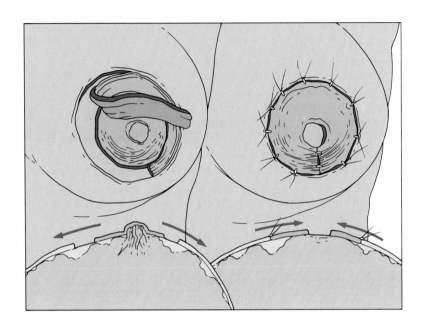

Reconstruction of the
Nipple-Areola Complex

Reconstruction of the nipple-areola complex is a minor procedure which gives the final touch to the breast reconstruction. Once volume and symmetry have been obtained, most patients (95% in our series) wish to have the areola and the nipple reconstructed. It is important that the areola be grafted onto a symmetrical breast. Any asymmetry will be more obvious after areola reconstruction.

Principles

The areola and nipple are best reconstructed with grafts. These grafts take well, considering that they are placed on skin which has been operated on at least twice, often irradiated, and which typically covers a large prosthesis. We have never had a total graft necrosis, and only exceptionally a partial loss.

The areola requires a full-thickness skin graft to imitate the color of the normal areola. Shaving and grafting from the surface of the normal areola led to scarring and depigmentation, and this practice has been abandoned. Our present choice is taking the external surface of the opposite areola if it is large enough. If not, we use tissue from the inner thigh.

The nipple should have some projection. This is obtained by grafting part of the opposite nipple or by creating a local flap.

Timing

The nipple-areola complex is better reconstructed 2 to 3 months after the breast reconstruction. Placement of the areola at the end of the breast procedure may displace it—usually upwards and laterally—by capsular contracture. This contracture displacement is impossible to correct without scarring the breast in the most visible center of the mound. If the reconstructed breast is not symmetrical, especially if there is asymmetry of position, it is best to correct this first. After a wait of 2 or 3 months until the breast has acquired its final shape, the areola can be reconstructed in a separate procedure.

Selection of Methods

Nipple-areola reconstruction is often disappointing for two reasons. The areolar pigmentation, as any other graft, tends to fade with time, particularly at the site of the scars. The nipple tends to retract and lose projection.

These observations lead to the following protocol: (1) the areola should be a full-thickness graft of a single piece of skin; and (2) the nipple should be created larger than needed to compensate for later retraction.

The methods chosen for reconstruction of the

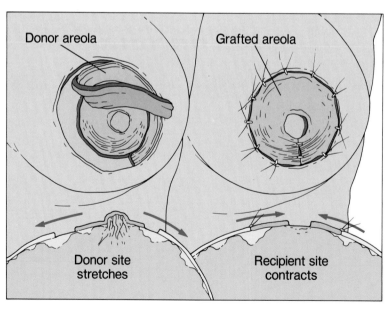

FIG. 8.1

areola and the nipple depend on several factors, most importantly the condition of the opposite breast and the wishes of the patient. Several questions need to be answered. Is the remaining areola large enough and the nipple protruding enough to share? What color is the areola? Does the patient have a scar on that side around the areola from a previous reduction or mastopexy? Is the breast big? (In that case the areola should be larger.) Some patients do not agree to have an operation on the sole sensitive area they still have.

The best donor site for the areola and the nipple is the opposite side, because it offers the same texture of skin. In some patients with a large areola and a flat nipple, the areola is shared for nipple-areola reconstruction. In others with a small areola and a large nipple *(Fig. 8.8)*, the nipple only will be shared. In other cases, the areola is reconstructed with a thigh graft *(Fig. 8.9)*. Nipple-areola reconstruction is usually performed with a local anesthetic as an outpatient procedure.

Surgical Technique

Areola from the Opposite Side

If the opposite areola is large enough and may be divided, a circle is drawn to determine the outer surface to be taken as a full-thickness graft *(Fig. 8.3)*. The diameter of the circle must be smaller than the diameter of the reconstructed areola, because some stretching is likely to occur on the donor site after suturing the areola to the surrounding breast skin. Suturing is done with a 4.0 nylon running suture left in place for 3 weeks. The grafted areola should be larger than needed because the graft will shrink *(Figs. 8.1, 8.2)*.

The graft for the reconstructed breast is chosen according to judgment and not to any measurement, for the skin over the reconstructed breast is often tighter than the other. A surface of 4 to 5 cm is de-epithelialized on the center of the breast cone. The graft is placed on this surface and sutured with 6.0 nylon, leaving a central surface of 1.5 cm uncovered. The preferred graft is made of one piece, with at most one suture placed in the lower part. Most donor areolae are not circular, and the graft is often irregular in diameter. Any excess graft should be cut from the narrowest part and kept for nipple reconstruction if needed.

During the first stage of breast reconstruction by subpectoral implantation with mastopexy of the opposite side in the patient shown in Fig. 8.2, the larger areola was not reduced. After 3 months, the outer surface of the areola was taken as a full-thickness skin graft, and a complementary mastopexy performed *(Fig. 8.3)*. The graft was used in

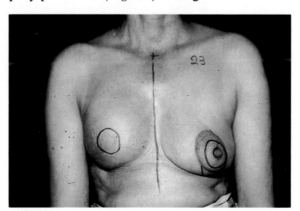

FIG. 8.2　　　　　　　　　　**FIG. 8.3**

one piece *(Fig. 8.4)*. The narrowest part of the graft was discarded, for it was not needed for nipple reconstruction, and the nipple was taken from the other side *(Fig. 8.5)*. After 3 years, the donor site was somewhat larger than the other side *(Figs. 8.6, 8.7)*. This could be expected because the graft was drawn a little too small *(Fig. 8.3)*.

Areola from the Thigh

If the opposite areola is small *(Fig. 8.8)* or the patient does not wish to have scars on that side, the best donor site choice for areola reconstruction is the thigh. With this method, it is easier to obtain the same diameter of both areolae. It should, however, be explained to the patient that the symmetry of the areolae is better if both are surrounded by scar as in sharing procedures.

When taking a graft from the thigh, several important points are considered. The scar should be hidden as much as possible. The donor site should be chosen according to the pigmentation of the opposite areola, remembering that the thigh skin

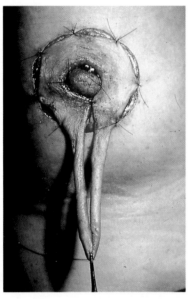

FIG. 8.4

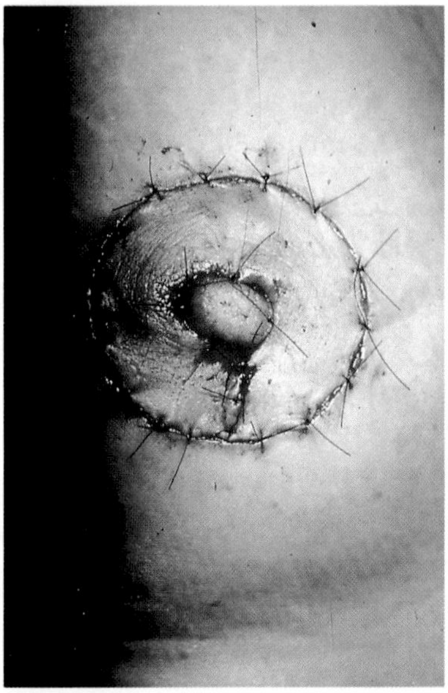

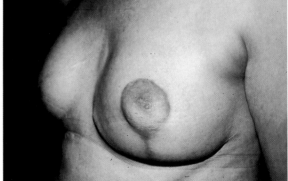

FIG. 8.5

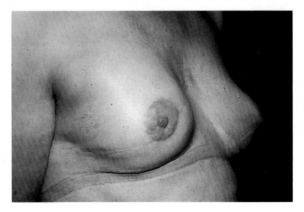

FIG. 8.6

FIG. 8.7

next to the labia is darker *(Figs. 8.9, 8.11).* If the donor site is hairy, some hair may grow on the graft, even if hair bulbs have been carefully cut from the graft.

A full-thickness graft is taken as an ellipse parallel to the thigh fold, its width being no less than the diameter of the areola. The extremities of the ellipse may be kept for nipple reconstruction.

Two months after breast reconstruction by sub-pectoral implantation and augmentation of the opposite breast by a subpectoral prosthesis, the reconstructed breast was still a little lower than the other *(Fig. 8.8).* A full-thickness graft was taken for areola reconstruction in the other part of the labia majora to match the opposite areola *(Fig. 8.9).* The donor nipple was sutured and the perineal skin and the opposite distal nipple were grafted *(Figs. 8.10, 8.11).*

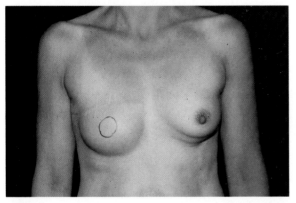

FIG. 8.8

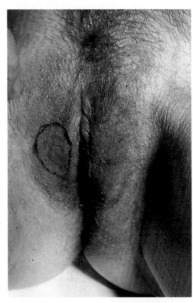

FIG. 8.9

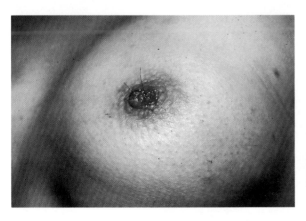

FIG. 8.10

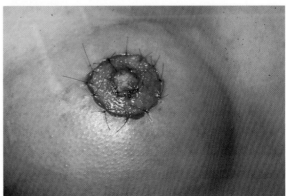

FIG. 8.11

Fourteen months later, the results are quite pleasing *(Fig. 8.12.A,B)*. The desired symmetry, diameter, and pigmentation have been achieved to the extent allowed by this procedure.

Nipple from the Opposite Nipple

Taking the opposite nipple as a free composite graft is the best choice. Obtaining a symmetrical result is not easy, however, because a nipple is a contractile organ and its length is difficult to judge.

Nipple sharing may be achieved by taking the outer part or the inferior half. Taking the outer nipple part by cutting parallel to the surface should be done carefully to avoid amputation *(Fig. 8.13)*. The raw surface may be sutured or, if more projection is desired, left to granulate and heal spontaneously. In this case, the donor nipple usually heals more slowly (2 to 3 weeks) than the recon-

structed one. Taking the inferior half of the nipple makes symmetry easier to achieve, but it produces less surface for covering the recipient area. This is why the first method is preferable.

Nipple from a Local Flap

Several methods of constructing a nipple from a local flap have been described, but few give a durable projection. Not only should the local flap survive, but also nourish a covering graft of the same skin as the rest of the areola.

After trying different techniques, we found that Olivari's technique, as described by Eder and Lejour,[1] yields the best results. His technique depends on finesse of performance as well as attention to surgical details and the quality of the recipient skin. If the place prepared for the nipple is scarred, a good result will not be obtained. After

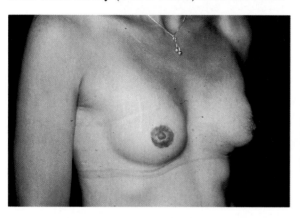

FIG. 8.12A

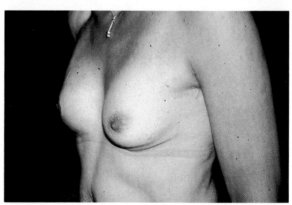

FIG. 8.12B

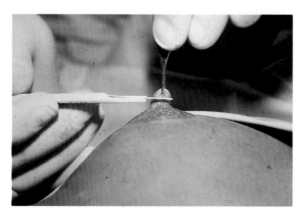

FIG. 8.13

the total surface for the nipple-areola complex has been de-epithelialized, a central 1.5-cm circle is incised in this surface. The incision is made perpendicular in the dermis and a little eccentric in the subcutaneous fat—as far as necessary (2 to 3 mm) to permit pulling the central flap gently outside the surface with small hooks *(Figs. 8.14, 8.15)*.

Fibrous adhesions, which might flatten the nipple, should be cut, keeping as many small vessels as possible in the flap. A running 4.0 nylon suture is used to place the nipple in the dermis of the areola and it is maintained for 3 weeks. When the sutures are tight, stretching of the areola will be prevented and the nipple will maintain its protrusion.

The areola is covered with the graft, leaving the center raw. A small piece of the same graft is cut to the size of the nipple and sutured on with 6.0 nylon. A piece of graft, about 15 mm × 2 mm, is cut from the same graft and placed as a collar around the shaft of the new nipple *(Figs. 8.16, 8.17)*. This collar graft should be slightly tight, but not enough to strangle the nipple. If it is too loose, it permits flattening of the nipple and the result is a flat nipple-areola complex of concentric circles.

No bolus dressing is necessary. The dressing is carefully made with petroleum jelly gauze, avoiding any compression on the nipple. The entire graft is covered with a thin gauze glued around the areola for 1 week.

After 1 week, the stitches are removed and a

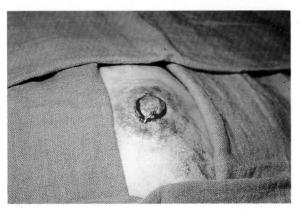

FIG. 8.14

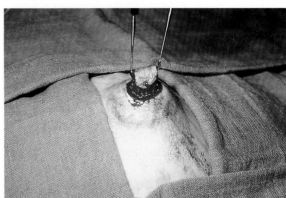

FIG. 8.15

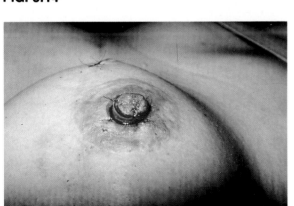

FIG. 8.16

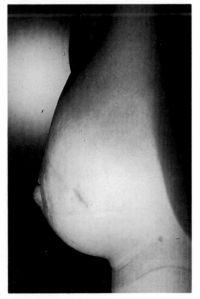

FIG. 8.17

new, similar dressing is put in place for another week. By that time the graft is usually completely healed. A small protective dressing which discharges pressure on the nipple is placed and changed regularly for the next 2 to 3 weeks. After the protective dressing is removed, the patient is encouraged to massage her graft with ointment like any other fresh graft.

The Skate Method

Determination of Nipple-Areola Position

Accurate location of the nipple-areola complex after breast reconstruction is of uppermost impor-tance. Malpositioning can give an unnatural appearance to an otherwise properly reconstructed breast *(Fig. 8.18).*

A simple, inexpensive aid useful in nipple-areola site determination is the disposable electrocardio-graphic electrode. The diameter of the electrode is easily adjusted to the size of the normal areola with the aid of scissors.

The patient should participate in the positioning of the future nipple-areola complex. Standing in front of a mirror, she and the surgeon make the final decision as to location. The ideal nipple location on the new breast may not be the measured location as determined by anatomic landmarks.

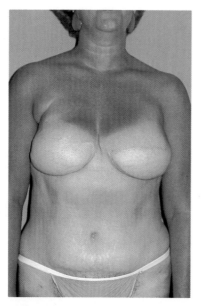

FIG. 8.18

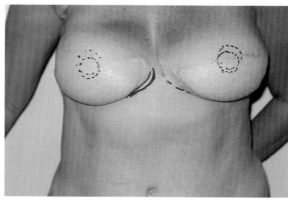

FIG. 8.19

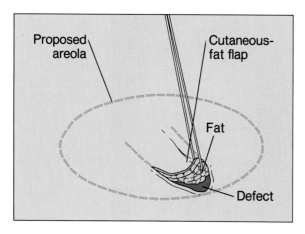

FIG. 8.20

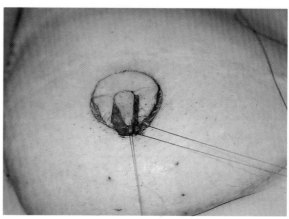

FIG. 8.21

The most reliable way of determining nipple position is by using Polaroid pictures. Even small malpositions are apparent in a picture *(Fig. 8.19)*.

Surgical Technique

The nipple flap is incised into the dermis *(Fig. 8.20)*, and then is elevated with a deep core of subcutaneous fat. The amount of fat taken with the flap is determined by the volume of the opposite nipple, but should be slightly larger to allow some shrinkage. Care must be taken at this point to protect the delicate blood supply entering from the subdermal plexus at the base of the flap *(Fig. 8.21)*.

The defect left by elevation of the dermal skin-fat flap is closed with 4.0 clear nylon sutures *(Fig. 8.22.A)*. This, in effect, traps the flap out of its bed.

Lateral dissection of the two skin flaps is performed cautiously *(Fig. 8.22.B)*. Dissection must be conservative and limited to the extent that nipple flap closure can be achieved without excessive tension. The flaps are wrapped around the raw surface and sutured into position *(Figs. 8.23, 8.24)*. The proposed areola is marked around the nipple. It is important that the areola be marked after the nipple is elevated and the defect closed to prevent distortion of the areola shape.

The proposed areola is de-epithelialized in a su-

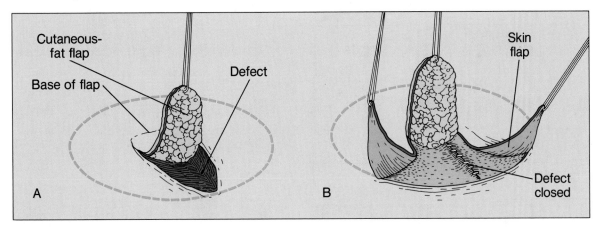

FIG. 8.22

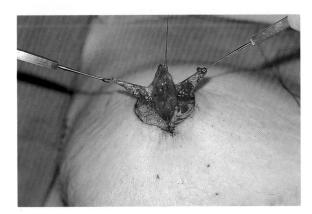

FIG. 8.23

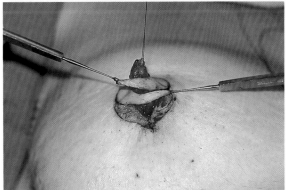

FIG. 8.24

perficial plane to avoid persistent bleeding that would jeopardize the graft *(Fig. 8.25)*.

Similarity in pigmentation and size with the contralateral areola is the goal. Grafts taken from the groin yield darkly pigmented skin with scant pubic hair. Closure of the groin donor defect is accomplished by a few deep absorbable sutures and a running subcuticular prolene suture.

The full-thickness graft is sutured to the dermal bed after a central slit is made to allow projection of the new nipple *(Figs. 8.26–8.28)*. A bolus dressing is not necessary. The graft is immobilized with sterile paper adhesive tape.

REFERENCES

1. Eder H, Lejour M: Reconstruction of the nipple-areola complex after radical mastectomy. *Acta Chir Belg 1980;79:147.*

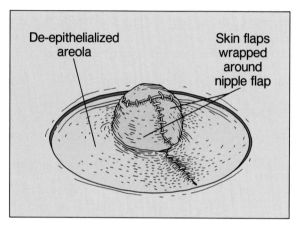

FIG. 8.25

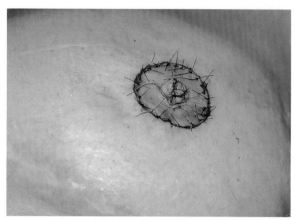

FIG. 8.26

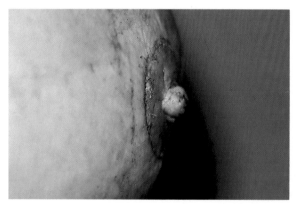

FIG. 8.27

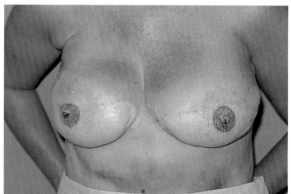

FIG. 8.28

CHAPTER · 9

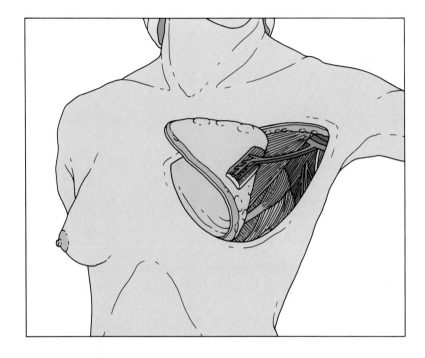

Special Problems and Secondary Corrections

INFRAMAMMARY CREASE

The chest wall skeleton is thought to be a valuable reference point for planning breast reconstructive procedures. Nonetheless, symmetry is the most important objective. When determining the inframammary sulcus, the patient should be placed in the standing and recumbent positions, and the location of the sulcus is to be compared with the opposite side. In patients with bilateral mastecto- mies, an arbitrary rib or interspace can be selected for a baseline. The skin markings, tattooed to the underlying muscle or periosteum of the rib with methilene blue, may help identify the proper level of the inferior dissection after making the skin incisions, but this method is not always reliable. In the TRAM flap method of reconstruction, the inframammary fold is maintained by dissecting a pocket down to it. The surgeon must not connect the abdominal dissection with the chest dissection,

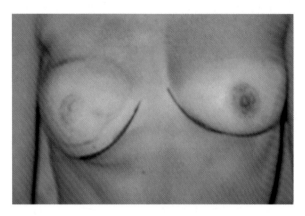

FIG. 9.1

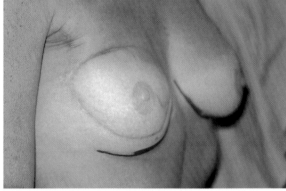

FIG. 9.2

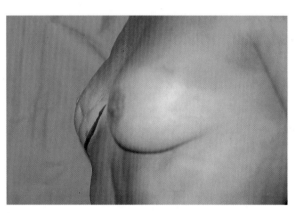

FIG. 9.3

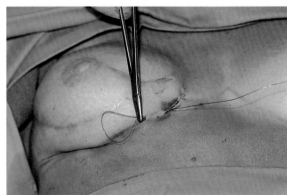

FIG. 9.4

except by a high tunnel through which the flap is passed. A bulging, medially from the muscle pedicle, will obscure the continuity of the inframammary fold, and it should be re-created secondarily.

TRAM Flap with Percutaneous Re-creation of the Inframammary Fold

Clinical Case

A 38-year-old woman had a lumpectomy and radiation for carcinoma of the right breast 2 years earlier. She underwent mastectomy with immediate TRAM flap reconstruction because of multiple suspicious areas around the nipple. *Figures 9.1–9.3* show a nicely reconstructed right breast, but an ill-defined inframammary fold on the medial aspect.

The inframammary fold was first marked with the patient sitting up. Polaroid pictures were taken, which served to demonstrate small asymmetries. Under local anesthesia, a 2-cm area superior and inferior to the marked fold was suctioned. Through small incisions, percutaneous sutures were placed connecting the deep tissues at the chest wall to the dermis, thus re-creating the inframammary fold *(Fig. 9.4). Figures 9.5–9.7* show the re-created fold.

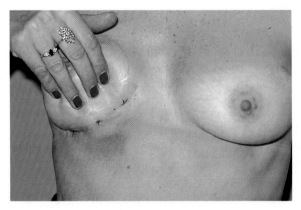

FIG. 9.5

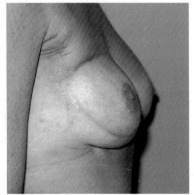

FIG. 9.6

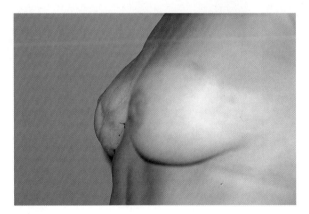

FIG. 9.7

Percutaneous Re-creation of the Inframammary Fold in Breast Reconstruction with Implant

Clinical Case

Figures 9.8–9.10 show a 40-year-old woman who had a modified radical mastectomy for stage II carcinoma of the right breast. She underwent a prophylactic left simple mastectomy with reconstruction of both breasts with Becker-type expander implants.

The upper abdominal skin was advanced to decrease the vertical skin deficit, and the inframammary fold was created percutaneously by anchoring the subdermal and subcutaneous tissue to the chest wall as the abdominal skin was lifted.

Figures 9.11–9.14 show the patient 8 months after breast reconstruction with Becker-type implants. The inframammary folds are satisfactory. When an inframammary fold is created by attaching the dermis to the chest wall in a patient with silicone implants, one always runs the risk that the possible capsular contracture will bring up the implant and the sulcus. When the sulcus is created secondarily, care must be exercised to avoid puncturing the implant.

SPECIAL RECONSTRUCTION PROBLEMS

Male Breast Carcinoma and Reconstruction

The incidence of carcinoma in the male breast is low. Most series report that carcinoma of the breast appears in approximately 1 man for every 100 women. In the United States the overall incidence of breast cancer in men is 0.7/100,000. The disease is very rare before the age of 30. A 5- to 10-year difference in the average age at diagnosis between men and women with breast cancer has been well documented. Recognition and treatment of the disease are often delayed.

Etiologic Considerations

The cause of breast cancer in men and women alike is unknown. Several factors have been implicated in its pathogenesis, including hormonal influences, heredity, gynecomastia, Klinefelter's syndrome, radiation, trauma, and bilharziasis.

Symptoms

In the vast majority of male breast cancer patients, the first symptom is a painless mass. Nipple discharge is an early symptom in as many as 15% of the patients. Bloody nipple discharge indicates

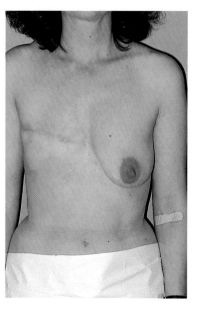

FIG. 9.8

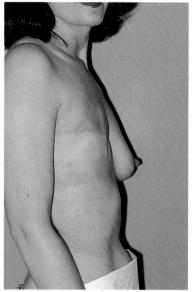

FIG. 9.9

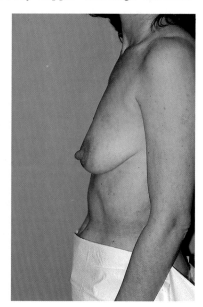

FIG. 9.10

malignancy in about 75% of the cases.[2] Other complaints include nipple or skin ulceration, nipple retraction, and an axillary mass.

Physical Findings

A subareolar mass is nearly always palpable. The tumor is generally hard, poorly defined, and not tender. Nipple retraction, nipple or skin ulceration, and skin fixation are present in about one third of patients.[11] Ipsilateral axillary lymph nodes are clinically positive in about 50% of men with breast cancer, although the clinical presence or absence of nodes does not correlate well with the pathologic findings in many cases.[2] There appears to be a slightly greater tendency for carcinoma to develop in the left breast rather than in the right one among men and women.

Staging

The staging of carcinoma of the breast in men is the same as in women. The determination should be completed before the initiation of definitive treatment.

Prognosis

Virtually all histologic types of breast cancer known to occur in women have been reported in men. As in the female, carcinomas arising from the ductal elements represent the most common type in men, whereas lobular carcinomas have been reported only rarely.[2] Estrogen and progesterone receptor activities have been measured in both male and female breast cancer patients. The prognosis is slightly poorer for men than for women, but not nearly as much as originally

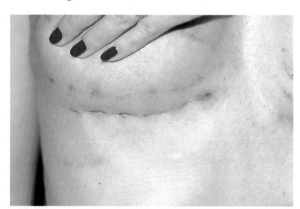

FIG. 9.11

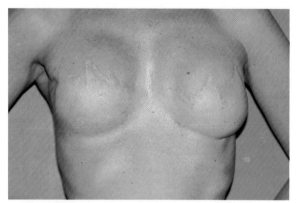

FIG. 9.12

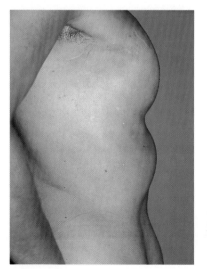

FIG. 9.13

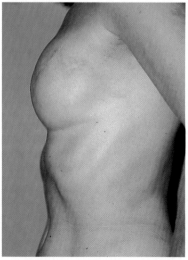

FIG. 9.14

thought. Although the survival rate of men with positive nodes seems to be slightly less than that for women, the overall survival is nearly equal if adjusted for age.[2]

Treatment

The treatment of choice for most types of male breast cancer is radical mastectomy. Skin grafting is nearly always considered necessary. Chemotherapy and hormonal manipulation also have been used as adjuvant therapy. Endocrine ablative procedures, as well as chemotherapy, have become the most important modalities in the treatment of metastatic disease.

Clinical Case

A 37-year-old man had a modified radical mastectomy on the left side for carcinoma of the breast. He was concerned about the considerable asymmetry of his chest *(Figs. 9.15, 9.16)*. The right breast was much larger than the left, inhibiting him from removing his shirt in public. There was a flattening of the upper portion of the chest, no well-defined inframammary fold, and the nipple had been removed.

Reconstruction of the breast in the male patient is unusual, but the same principles applied to the reconstruction of the female breast should be kept

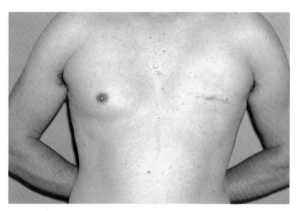

FIG. 9.15

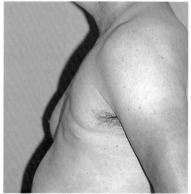

FIG. 9.16

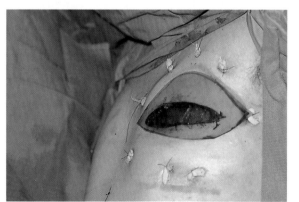

FIG. 9.17

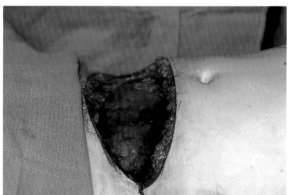

FIG. 9.18

in mind. Our reconstruction plan in this patient was to advance the upper abdominal skin, to recreate the inframammary fold, and to fill the upper chest concavity with a sandwich dermal graft (with minimal or no fat) obtained from the lower abdomen. The nipple was to be reconstructed in a second-stage procedure.

The transverse incision was reopened on the left side *(Fig. 9.17)*. The upper abdominal flap was undermined for a considerable distance, and then advanced superiorly to provide additional skin. An inframammary fold was created with deep sutures approximating subcutaneous tissue to the intercostal spaces at the same level as the contralateral one. This is important in creating symmetry.

The patient had a considerable concavity at the upper portion of the chest, which was repaired with a sandwich dermal graft taken from the lower abdomen. *Figure 9.18* shows the defect in the suprapubic region after a large ellipse of skin was obtained.

After de-epithelializing and defatting, the sandwich dermal fat graft was fashioned to fill the chest defect *(Fig. 9.19)*. The fat side was approximated to the fat side of the graft, and traction-type sutures were placed to maintain the sandwiched dermis under tension. The sutures, left long, were threaded into a Keith needle and passed percutaneously at a distance to maintain the graft maximally stretched.

Figure 9.20 shows the satisfactory correction of the upper chest concavity. *Figure 9.21* shows the

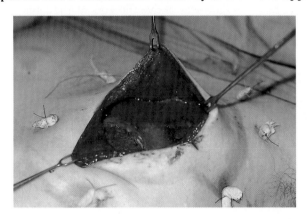

FIG. 9.19

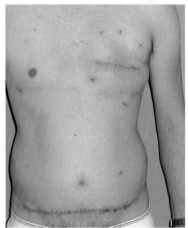

FIG. 9.20

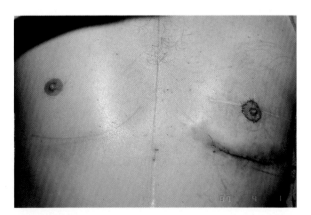

FIG. 9.21

patient after nipple-areola reconstruction and re-creation of the inframammary fold. The results, 18 months postoperatively, are revealed in *Figures 9.22 and 9.23.*

TRAM FLAP AFTER LATISSIMUS DORSI MUSCLE FAILURE

The use of the latissimus dorsi myocutaneous flap with an implant offers a good and reliable option for reconstruction. However, the method is not entirely satisfactory when performed in an obese patient or in patients with a large contralateral breast. In the case of obese patients, asymmetry is the reason for the dissatisfaction of patient and surgeon alike. Because a silicone implant has to be used, the newly reconstructed breast is rounded and has a certain degree of capsular contracture, bulges superiorly, and does not match the usually large and ptotic contralateral breast.

Clinical Case

A 47-year-old woman had a modified radical mastectomy on the left side for adenocarcinoma *(Fig. 9.24).* She underwent a latissimus dorsi myocutaneous flap breast reconstruction which was complicated with capsule development, extrusion of the implant, and infection. Correction attempts by the insertion of skin expanders were unsuccessful, resulting in the expander extruding through the medial aspect of the wound.

The abdomen, which was almost like an apron over the suprapubic area, showed considerable dimpling and striae. She had a well-healed right transverse scar at the level of the umbilicus, as well as in the suprapubic region. *Figure 9.25* shows a stellate scar above the area of the latissimus dorsi donor flap.

The ipsilateral TRAM flap was chosen because the patient had a transverse scar at the level of the

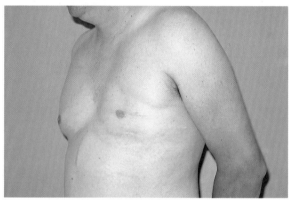

FIG. 9.23

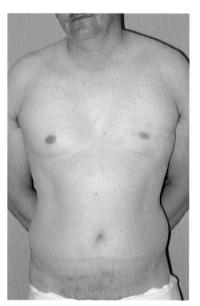

FIG. 9.22

umbilicus on the contralateral right side. The upper incision of the flap was outlined approximately 4 cm above the umbilicus and down to the pubis. The entire rectus muscle was freed and used.

The reconstruction plan was to use the de-epithelialized latissimus island flap to fill the subclavicular hollow and restore fullness for the axillary concavity. The breast mound itself was achieved by the ipsilateral TRAM flap, which had to be turned approximately 90°, placing the left extent of the flap to correspond to the inframammary line.

Improvement was achieved in the abdominal contour and breast *(Figs. 9.26–9.28).* The results, 1 month after nipple and areola reconstruction on

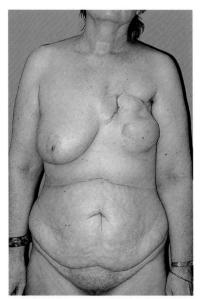

FIG. 9.24

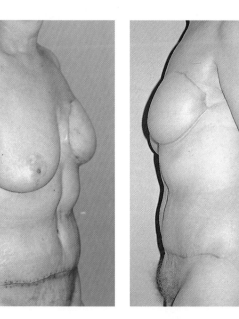

FIG. 9.25

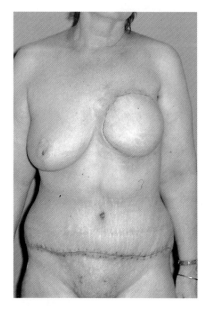

FIG. 9.26   FIG. 9.27   FIG. 9.28

the left breast and mastopexy on the right breast, are shown in *Figures 9.29* and *9.30*.

CONGENITAL BREAST ASYMMETRY

Poland's Anomaly

Definitions

Poland's syndrome, also called Poland's anomaly, consists of a unilateral absence of the sternocostal head of the pectoralis major and symbrachydactyly of the ipsilateral hand. Other frequent manifestations include hypoplasia of the breast and nipple on the same side. Isolated absence of the pectoralis major muscle with breast hypoplasia is a variant of the Poland's defect. In Sprengel's deformity, one or both scapulae can be hypoplastic or congenitally elevated, with the lower angle turned toward the spine. This deformity can be an isolated condition, but it is frequently seen together with Poland's anomaly. This anomaly comes in different variations and degrees of severity, ranging from hypoplasia of the breast with only partial absence of the lower portion of the pectoralis major muscle and an intact clavicular portion to the total absence of the pectoralis major muscle as well as the breast.

Pathogenic Hypothesis

In the patient with Poland's anomaly, the upper girdle may have multiple anomalies and in various combinations. These variations include, aside from the absence of the pectoralis major and breast hypoplasia, defects of the terminal transverse limbs, and the Sprengel, Klippel-Feil, and Möbius anomalies. These conditions may share a common pathogenesis; the causative effect has been suggested to be an interruption of the blood supply to the major embryonic structures which are supplied by the subclavicular arteries and their branches. The specific combination of birth defects would depend on the location, extent, and timing of the disruptive event.

Figure 9.31 lists the possible causes for interruption or reduction of blood in the subclavicular arteries and their branches.

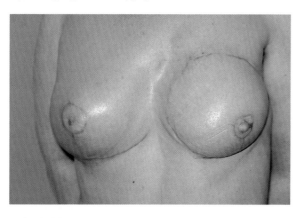

FIG. 9.29

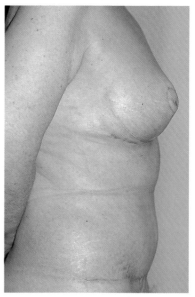

FIG. 9.30

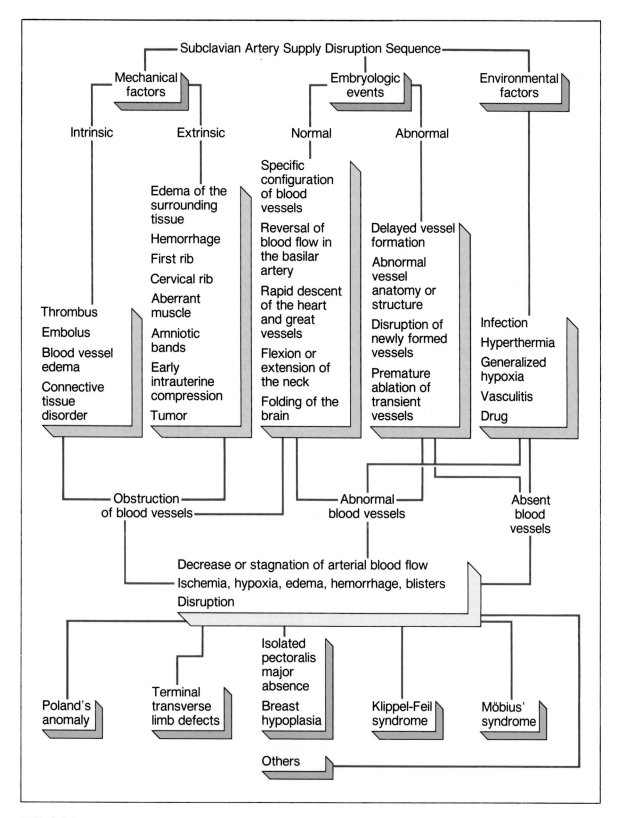

FIG. 9.31

Some clinical evidence supports the vascular theory of pathogenesis. In his original article describing the anomaly, Poland[10] noted that the autopsy revealed very small thoracic arteries in the affected side. Bouvet et al[1] studied eight children with Poland's anomaly using impedance plethysmography. The tests showed marked decrease in arterial blood flow velocities in the affected sides, suggesting hypoplasia of the subclavicular artery. Additional indirect evidence for a vascular etiology comes from the clinical observation of increased occurrence of dextrocardia in individuals with Poland's anomaly on the left side. Isolated dextrocardia occurs in approximately 1 in 30,000 newborn infants. A literature review reveals that 7 of 73 (9.6%) of infants with Poland's anomaly had dextrocardia. The apparently significant increase of this defect suggests an underlying problem in cardiovascular development.[3-5,7-9]

Treatment

Because Poland's syndrome is seen in varying degrees of severity, each case must be analyzed individually. Remarks here will be limited to corrections of the anterior chest wall as well as breast underdevelopment.

Severe Deformity

Patients with severe deformity usually show an absence of the pectoralis major muscle, which produces a subclavicular hollow and flattening of the anterior chest. The breast tissue is underdeveloped, and the nipple and areola are smaller. Upon extending the arm, the anterior axillary fold is absent, but the posterior fold formed by the latissimus dorsi muscle is usually intact.

Clinical Case

A 13-year-old girl presented with Poland's syndrone on the left side, specifically, underdevelopment of the breast and the nipple (Figs. 9.32, 9.33). Absence of the pectoralis muscle was not apparent because of her mild obesity. Because there was no pectoralis major muscle, treatment was begun with insertion of a skin expander in the subcutaneous plane. The expander was inflated, percutaneously, at weekly intervals (Fig. 9.34). Use of an IV pole facilitates slow and continuous injection. Three months after insertion of the expander, the patient's breasts were fairly symmetric, although she had developed striae on the site of the expander (Figs. 9.35, 9.36). Expansion was continued at intervals to keep up with the growing right breast. After puberty, we will consider removing the expander and exchanging it for a permanent implant.

Male Patients

In men, the objective for correction of Poland's syndrome is to fill the subclavicular hollow and to correct the flattening on the anterior chest (Figs. 9.37–9.39). If possible, the underdeveloped nipple and areola are lowered.

Transposition of the latissimus dorsi muscle has been advocated for this defect. The muscle is transposed as a pendulum, if necessary, dividing

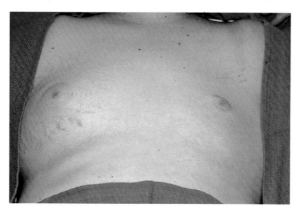

FIG. 9.32

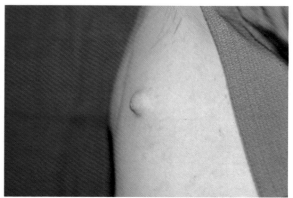

FIG. 9.33

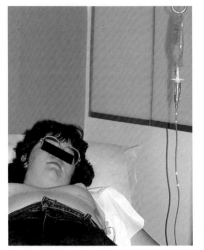

FIG. 9.34

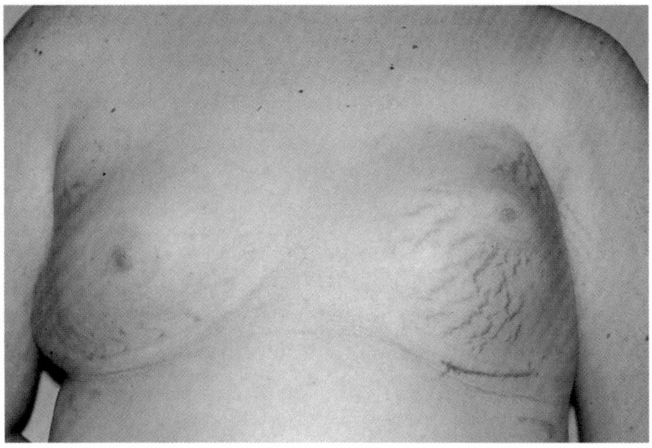

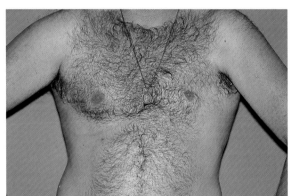

FIG. 9.35

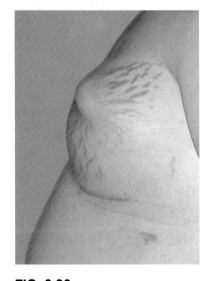

FIG. 9.36

FIG. 9.37

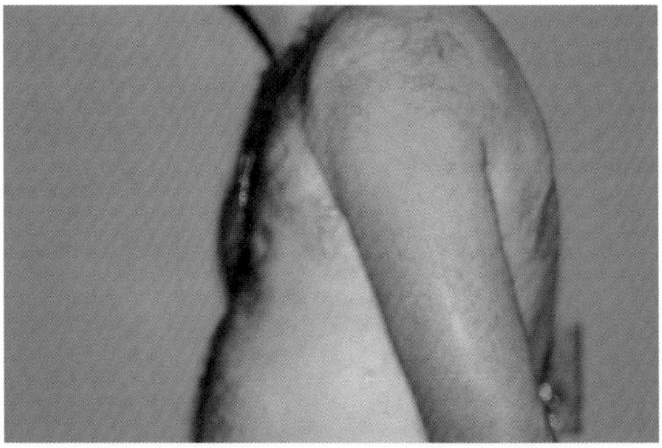

FIG. 9.38

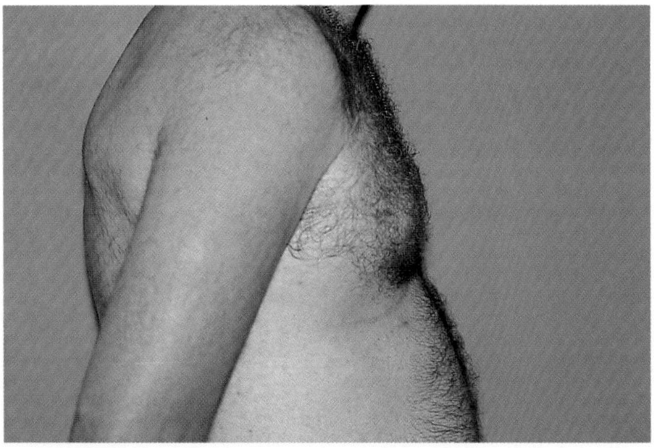

FIG. 9.39

not only its origin but also its insertion along the humerus. The muscle is repositioned at a more anterior place in the humerus, similar to where the pectoralis major muscle inserts. Although this is the most attractive solution to the problem, it has not received thorough and long-term evaluation. Long-term follow-up of two of our patients has shown that the transposed latissimus dorsi muscle is inadequate in thickness or bulk to correct the subclavicular hollow as well as the flattening of the anterior chest wall. In addition, the smaller nipple and areola have not been improved. An added disadvantage is the loss of the posterior axillary fold.

Preformed and custom-made silicone implants have been used to correct the deformity. The disadvantage of using an implant is that it will form a capsule, and, although the edges may be feathered, they are still noticeable as well as palpable. Even if they are anchored to the periosteum of the clavicle, most implants will in time descend and drop, re-creating the subclavicular hollow.

While the use of a skin expander may be an acceptable solution for the correction of Poland's anomaly in men, no reports of this technique appear in published medical studies, nor have we used this technique.

Female Patients

The objective of correction in Poland's syndrome in the female patient is not only to correct the subclavicular hollow, but also to match the opposite breast which may vary in size as well as pendulousness.

The simplest method and one that has achieved acceptable results is the use of a skin expander, particularly if it is inserted at puberty and is in place as the breast develops. For reasons that are not clear, the breast, as well as the nipple and areola, seem to descend as well as to expand, and may approximate or match the contralateral normal breast. The expander may not fill the subclavicular

defect, but the defect may be ameliorated by a projection obtained with the skin expander or with the permanent silicone implant. A custom-made implant with an extension to fill the subclavicular hollow may be tried. The edges will still be evident and palpable, and eventually it may drop from its original placement. The degree of satisfaction with custom-made implants is variable.

Although the use of the transposed latissimus dorsi muscle and an implant has been advocated, it has not received long-term evaluation. If the latissimus dorsi muscle is to be transferred anteriorly, we suggest to do it through an oblique incision in the axilla, approximately 10-cm long and located at the anterior border of the muscle. Although the dissection of the muscle is a more tedious and time consuming procedure, it can be done with the aid of fiberoptic retractors.

De-epithelialized TRAM Flap

Hartrampf[6] has corrected severe Poland's anomalies with the use of a patterned de-epithelialized flap from the infraumbilical area transferred onto the chest wall. This technique is similar to breast reconstruction with a transverse island flap. He has obtained impressive corrections even in young, relatively thin, athletic women. Closure of the abdomen was obtained in all cases, with moderate but acceptable tension.

TRAM FLAP TO CORRECT SUBCUTANEOUS MASTECTOMY—PERSISTENT PROBLEMS

The cosmetic result of a subcutaneous mastectomy is not always acceptable. Complications can be classified according to the time of occurrence. Early complications include necrosis of the nipple and/or necrosis of the skin flaps with resulting exposure of the prosthesis. Severe scarring and skin wrinkling inevitably follow these complications. Even if the breast reconstruction is delayed after subcutaneous mastectomy, the remaining skin usually becomes so wrinkled and the nipple so malpositioned that the final cosmetic result is jeopardized. Late complications include implant displacement, wrinkling, persistent mastodynia, and severe capsular contracture.

When subcutaneous mastectomy complications arise after silicone implants have failed, the rectus abdominis myocutaneous flap procedure provides an adequate breast mound without the use of a prosthesis. The overlying skin that is irreparably damaged can be excised. The de-epithelialized flap is placed beneath the capsule or at the subcutaneous plane.

Clinical Case

Figures 9.40–9.42 show a 37-year-old woman who had infiltrated ductal adenocarcinoma of the right breast 9 years earlier. The patient underwent a modified right radical mastectomy with reimplantation of the nipple and a prophylactic subcutaneous mastectomy on the left side. Reconstruction of both breasts was accomplished with the use of silicone implants. Three years after the mastectomy she developed recurrent carcinoma in the same place where the primary tumor had been. The recurrent tumor was treated by local resection and radiation therapy to the inner quadrants of the right breast and to the internal mammary chain.

The left side shows a subcutaneous mastectomy with well-healed scars and capsular contracture which has elevated the breast, making it prominent at the subclavicular level. The nipple has been grafted high and has no projection. Besides asymmetry, the patient complained of severe pain and discomfort, which we thought was due to the capsular contracture.

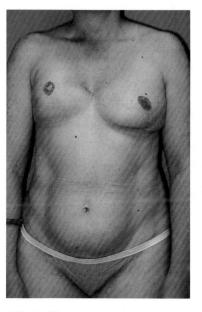
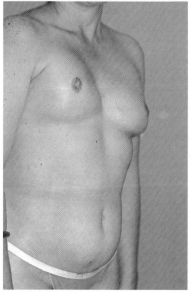
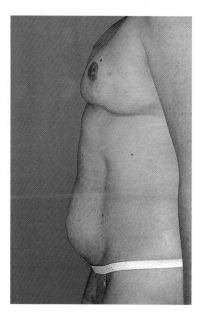

FIG. 9.40   **FIG. 9.41**   **FIG. 9.42**

The bilateral TRAM flap was performed; the skin flap was divided in the midline from the umbilicus toward the pubis and elevated with the entire rectus muscle to carry the ipsilateral island flap *(Figs. 9.43–9.45)*. The submammary incisions were opened bilaterally and the silicone implants removed. The right pectoralis major muscle had been previously resected at the time of the local recurrence.

The ipsilateral flaps were de-epithelialized, anchored with the dermis side down toward the chest, and supported with sutures. More tissue was used on the right side.

The restoration was good in the upper part but deficient in inferior projection, requiring two additional procedures for correction.

As shown in *Fig. 9.46,* the inframammary fold on the right side is not clearly delineated and bulges along the costal margin, whereas on the left side the inframammary fold has only partial definition. The first additional correction was accomplished by opening the incision at the submammary folds. Both rectus abdominis muscle pedicles were identified and divided along the costal margin. The muscle and the underlying fat were freed from the chest wall and turned under to project the cone. The second additional procedure consisted in re-creating the inframammary fold percutaneously with sutures connecting the subcutaneous tissue to the chest wall. The fullness along the cos-

tal margin was further corrected with suction-assisted lipectomy performed at the same time.

Figures 9.47–9.49 show the patient 1 month following the creation of submammary folds. The breasts appear to be quite soft and symmetric. A secondary correction of the right nipple-areola position is necessary. Other than excising the nipple and areola, closing the defect, and making a new nipple-areola, little else can be done.

SUBCLAVICULAR (HOLLOW) DEFECT

A depression just below the clavicle is the most annoying deformity for a patient, often surpassing concern for the loss of the breast mound. The reason is simple, for a breast mound can be camouflaged with a prosthesis, external or otherwise, whereas the patient with a subclavicular hollow is unable to wear any clothing cut below the clavicles.

Occurrence

Fortunately, the severe deformity produced by removing the active pectoralis major muscle (including its clavicular portion) is rare today because of the fewer Halsted-type mastectomies performed. However, mild concavities are often seen following even modified mastectomies. These concavities occur whenever the takeoff of the breast is rel-

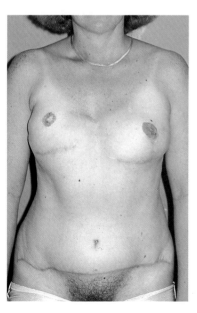

FIG. 9.43

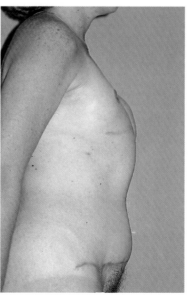

FIG. 9.44

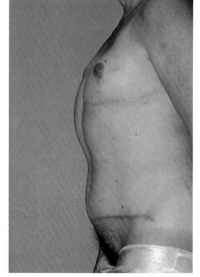

FIG. 9.45

atively high. As the surgeon elevates thin flaps to the level of the clavicle and removes the breast from the pectoralis major muscle, a flat surface is left which at times is concave when compared with the other side. The difference will be apparent even after a standard reconstruction with implants.

A concavity is also seen when the pectoralis major muscle has atrophied because of injury to the medial or lateral pectoral nerves. Such injuries may occur during the modified mastectomy if the surgeon transects the origin of the pectoralis minor muscle in an effort to gain access to the highest lymph node. The atrophy of the muscle is usually segmental and more apparent in the unreconstructed breast.

Treatment

Mild deformities in patients who have undergone modified mastectomies and who have a small normal contralateral breast with a low takeoff are easily camouflaged after reconstruction with the use of implants. Care should be used, however, not to place the reconstructive implant too high in an effort to camouflage the concavity, because excessive subclavicular bulging is just as much of a concern, or more so, than the hollowness.

For more severe defects, the methods advocated for treatment include use of preformed or patterned silicone implants, dermal or fascial grafts, the latissimus dorsi muscle (alone), or the latissi-

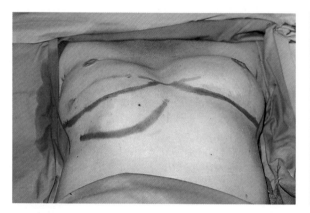

FIG. 9.46

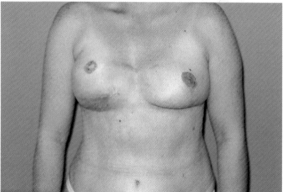

FIG. 9.47

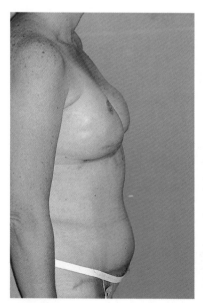

FIG. 9.48

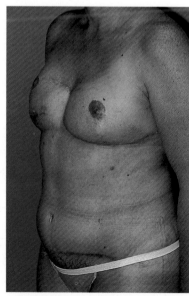

FIG. 9.49

mus dorsi myocutaneous flap with a de-epithelialized patterned skin island.

Preformed Silicone Implants

The use of preformed silicone implants appears to be an attractive idea. From a pattern of the subclavicular defect, an implant could be constructed exactly to correct the problem area. Unfortunately, even though the implant may be anchored to the clavicle, it still has a tendency to drop. In every case the implant forms a capsule, and the edges are palpable and easily seen. The results have been unsatisfactory to most patients, and this method is recommended only for special circumstances.

Dermal or Fascial Grafts

For relatively mild defects, a pattern of the shape and size of the defect can be obtained and a sandwiched dermal graft constructed. Our use of this method in three cases gave satisfactory results.

Surgical Technique

The pattern of the defect is outlined on x-ray paper. For the donor site, we suggest using the mid-buttock area instead of the gluteal crease or the suprapubic area. Particularly in young pa-

tients, the mid-buttock area provides a relatively thick dermis, and the scar is easily covered and does not produce a defect in the gluteal crease *(Fig. 9.50)*. The pattern is converted into an ellipse to facilitate wound closure. Usually a two-layer sandwich dermal graft is necessary. The bilateral ellipse taken from the mid-buttocks is de-epithelialized as thin as possible. The remaining dermis, with a minimal amount of subcutaneous tissue, is removed from the buttocks. The donor sites are closed primarily without any undermining *(Fig. 9.50)*. The dermal grafts are opposed to each other, "fat to fat," after adequate defatting. The edges are sutured with fine nylon and the ends of the sutures are left long.

The mastectomy scar is partially opened, and the overlying skin is freed from the pectoralis major muscle about 1 or 2 cm beyond the borders of the defect. The sandwiched dermal graft is then properly oriented. Most of the time, even if the defect is not in the exact form of an ellipse, all that is needed is to trim one end or the other before the graft is inserted. To facilitate the proper placement of the graft, the long sutures are threaded through a straight Keith needle. With the aid of a fiberoptic retractor, the two sutures are then passed at a distance, about 2 to 3 cm beyond the defect, and are tied over a bolster. By passing both sutures through the same hole, one avoids necrosis on the overlying skin. An effort is made to maintain the

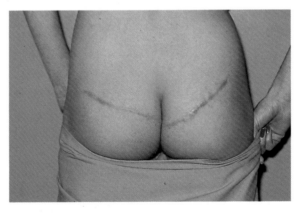

FIG. 9.50

sandwich dermal graft as stretched out as possible. Suturing the dermis to the underlying pectoralis fascia or to the overlying dermis of the skin flap is not necessary and is definitely much more difficult. Revascularization is faster if the sandwich graft is placed dermis toward the undersurface of the skin flap and also dermis toward the pectoralis fascia. This technique also ensures the survival of both layers without any loss of substance.

After the sutures have been tied at a distance over bolsters, a pressure dressing is placed over the skin covering the dermal sandwich graft, which is maintained for approximately 1 week.

Latissimus Dorsi Muscle Camouflage

The use of the latissimus dorsi muscle to camouflage the loss of the pectoralis major muscle and to correct the subclavicular hollow has also been proposed. In practice, however, this correction has not worked out because the muscle is not as thick as the pectoralis major muscle; when it is transferred, a certain amount of atrophy may be expected. Even in cases when the latissimus dorsi muscle has been folded to make it thicker and thus allow a better camouflage of the subclavicular defect, the coverage has not been sufficient over the long term because of muscle atrophy and lack of bulk. Consequently, this method is advisable for use in relatively mild defects or when one needs to cover an implant with additional muscle.

De-epithelialized Latissimus Dorsi Myocutaneous Flap

The most satisfactory method for correction of the subclavicular defect is the de-epithelialized latissimus dorsi myocutaneous flap.

Figure 9.51 shows a patient who had a Halsted-type mastectomy resulting in a subclavicular hollow extending along the lateral border of the sternum. The patient wanted a match of the opposite breast. Specifically, she did not want a mastopexy or the insertion of a silicone implant in her normal breast.

The subclavicular hollow was corrected with a patterned de-epithelialized myocutaneous latissimus dorsi flap. For the breast mound, a contralateral upper rectus flap was used. *Figure 9.51* shows the patient preoperatively, an outline of the subclavicular defect extending above the oblique mastectomy scar toward the clavicle and along the lateral border of the sternum. This triangle was transferred to the back, indicating the island of skin over the latissimus dorsi muscle. The latissimus dorsi muscle with the overlying skin was de-epithelialized and transferred toward the chest *(Fig. 9.52)*. The muscle was freed completely, leaving it attached to its insertion and also its vascular pedicle. The bulge along the anterior axillary line was thus avoided. The de-epithelialized dermis was sutured to the clavicle and along the lateral border of the sternum, overcorrecting the subclav-

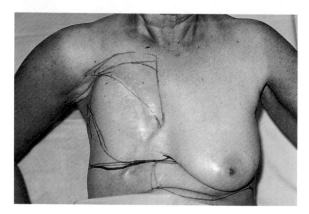

FIG. 9.51

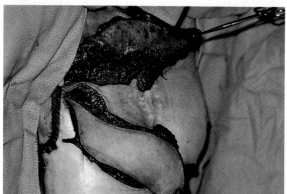

FIG. 9.52

icular defect. At the same time, the upper rectus flap was transferred to the contralateral side to allow reconstruction of the breast mound, which also required simultaneous insertion of a silicone implant.

Figures 9.53, 9.54 show the patient postoperatively. The subclavicular hollow is completely corrected, including a nice "teardrop" result simulating the opposite side.

REFERENCES

1. Bouvet JP, Leveque D, Bernetieres F, et al: Vascular origin of Poland syndrome? *Eur J Pediatr 1978;128:17.*
2. Crichlow RW: Carcinoma of the male breast. *Surg Gynecol Obstet 1972;134:1011.*
3. David TJ: Nature and etiology of the Poland anomaly. *N Engl J Med 1972;10:487.*
4. Goldberg MJ, Mazzei RJ: Poland syndrome: a concept of pathogenesis based on limb bud embriology. *Birth Defects 1977;13:103.*
5. Hanka SS: Dextrocardia associated with Poland's syndrome (letter). *J Pediatr 1975; 86(2):312.*
6. Hartrampf CR Jr: *Transverse Abdominal Island Flap Technique for Breast Reconstruction After Mastectomy.* Baltimore, University Park Press, 1984.
7. Hedge HR, Shokeir MHK: Posterior shoulder girdle abnormalities with absence of pectoralis major muscle. *Am J Med Genet 1982;13:285.*
8. Ireland DCR, Takayama N, Flatt AE: Poland's syndrome. *J Bone Joint Surg 1976;58(1):52.*
9. McGillivray BC, Lowry RB: Poland syndrome in British Columbia: incidence and reproductive experience of affected persons. *Am J Med Genet 1977;1:65.*
10. Poland A: Deficiency of the pectoral muscles. Reported by Mr. Alfred Poland. *Guy's Hosp Rep 1841;6:191.*
11. Scheike O: Male breast cancer. *Acta Pathol Microbiol Scand 1975;251(suppl):13.*

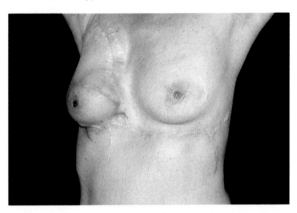

FIG. 9.53

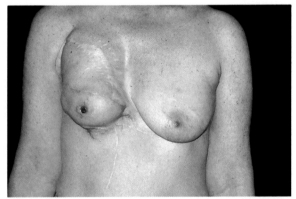

FIG. 9.54

CHAPTER · 10

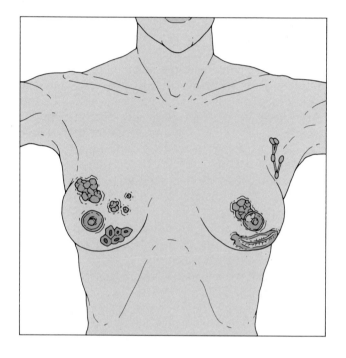

Breast Carcinoma: Treatment and Reconstruction of Local Recurrences or Postradiation Ulcers

LOCAL RECURRENCES

Local recurrence after surgical treatment of mammary cancer may occur within the scars, the chest wall or, rarely, the axilla. Local recurrence may be a sign of systemic dissemination—in more than 90% of such recurrences, systemic disease is present. It is accepted that these recurrences rarely emanate from tumor cells left behind at the time of operation or from those surviving radiation therapy. From a biological point of view, they should be regarded as metastases and treated accordingly.

Most large studies show that 75% of local recurrences will be diagnosed within 2 years following the initial surgical treatment. In isolated cases, however, local recurrences and distant metastases have been noted 30 years or longer after the primary treatment. *Figure 10.1* shows a local recurrence in the chest wall 5 years after a radical mastectomy without radiation.

A local recurrence in the chest wall often can be easily diagnosed as painless lumps with adjacent adherence within or under the skin. Needle and/or excisional biopsy and histopathology will rapidly confirm the diagnosis. Plans for therapy and reconstruction require a complete workup for possible disseminated disease and the involvement of surrounding tissues, such as muscles, ribs, or the brachial plexus. *Figure 10.2* shows metastases in the internal mammary chain. It should be noted that reconstruction does not seem to mask or hide local recurrences, because they tend to occur at the subcutaneous or skin level, which is easily palpable.

POSTRADIATION ULCERS

Any ionizing radiation treatment will cause damage to skin and underlying structures, varying from frank ulceration to microscopic changes. The changes start in the small blood vessels as radiation-induced obliterative endarteritis and progress to fibrosis of surrounding tissues. In addition, direct damage to cells includes chromosomal changes that prevent normal cell recovery and reproduction. Local lymphedema, increased hyalinization of elastic fibers, and thrombosis of arterioles and venulae, over time, cause nutritional disturbances and hypoxia in local tissues. These effects accumulate, resulting in delays and failure of superficial ulcerations to heal. The appearance of these visible lesions is dependent on the radiation dose, type, and modality of application. Modern radiotherapeutic techniques spare or minimize damage to the skin.

Figure 10.3 shows extensive radionecrosis of the chest following high-voltage radiotherapy. This type of lesion is seen rarely at the present time. Other less frequently seen sequelae of radiation include radionecrosis of the ribs or clavicle, fibrosis of the pleura and pulmonary parenchyma, and damage and fibrosis around the brachial plexus. Lymphedema of the arm with reduced mobility is another sequelae, more likely to occur in a patient who has also had an axillary dissection.

TREATMENT

We favor surgical excision to manage isolated local recurrences. Radiation therapy is a second-level option, not indicated in postradiation recurrences. When distant metastases are present, an excision of a local recurrence to reduce the tumor mass may still be helpful, even though the cancer may have spread systemically.

The radiodermatitis, radionecrosis, and painful radiation ulcers should be excised and replaced by well-vascularized tissue, preferably muscle and smooth mobile skin. Even if survival time is not increased, this treatment will dramatically improve the patient's quality of life.

Contraindications for surgical intervention are a poor prognosis from the underlying tumor and the patient's poor general condition.

Surgical Technique

Local recurrence or radiation sequelae should be treated surgically as primary tumors, with adequate margins, peripherally and in depth. If indicated, ribs, part of the sternum, or even the complete chest wall may have to be resected.

Preliminary biopsies are not essential in patients with frank postradiation ulcers, because the treatment will be the same (wide excision) and because of the difficulty of pathologic interpretation. The pathologist is likely to read the biopsy as "chronic ulceration, tumor cannot be ruled out." What is important in the treatment of a postradiation ulcer, however, is that the margins of excision should extend to include not only the ulcer but also all the surrounding skin affected by radiation. This skin is usually pigmented, telangiectatic, and without skin appendages. In short, all the area encompassed by the portal of radiation should be excised.

The defect, which is usually large, should be covered with a flap which brings in its own blood supply, preferably muscle with skin, or omentum. If the underlying ribs have been resected, stabilization of the chest wall is easily obtained by suturing a layer of polypropylene mesh.

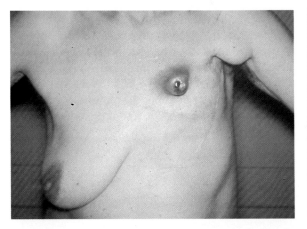

FIG. 10.1

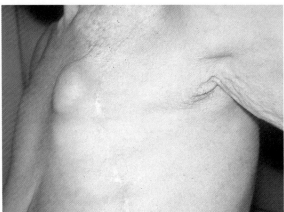

FIG. 10.2

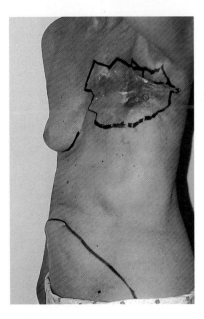

FIG. 10.3

Figures 10.4, 10.5 show an anterior and posterior view of an extensive resection of the chest wall for a local recurrence of breast carcinoma. Most large defects must be covered immediately by well-vascularized flaps, such as a myocutaneous latissimus or TRAM flap, or with omentum.

With standard irradiation dosages and delivery techniques, changes on the chest wall should be minimal and should not be a contraindication for TRAM flap use. The contralateral pedicle has been used most often in patients with an irradiated chest. The ipsilateral irradiated internal thoracic vessels, however, have also been used as the pedicle with few problems. In one patient with postmediastinal irradiation for Hodgkin's disease, a unilateral TRAM flap which appeared dusky was salvaged by adding the revascularization of the in-ferior epigastric artery and vein to the thoracodorsal vessels ("supercharging the flap").

Other variations in flap design include placing the flap higher on the abdomen. In most cases, two vascular pedicles are used to cover one side of the chest. We recommend this technique and feel it is the safest for postradiation chest ulcers *(Fig. 10.3)*.

Clinical Case

A 64-year-old patient with a left radical mastectomy was seen 11 years after postoperative radiotherapy (5,000 rads). Changes in the left chest wall include a large postradiation ulcer and an extensive chest defect *(Fig. 10.3)*. *Figure 10.6* shows the defect following excision of the radiation ulcer and surrounding tissue. *Figure 10.7* reveals the double

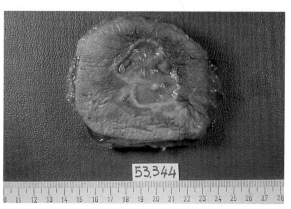

FIG. 10.4

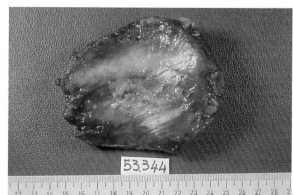

FIG. 10.5

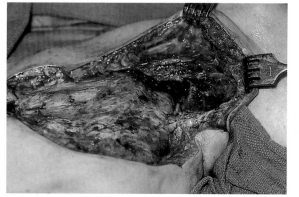

FIG. 10.6

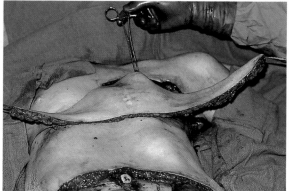

FIG. 10.7

pedicle TRAM flap necessary for coverage of the large chest defect, and *Figure 10.8* shows the immediate postoperative view with the flap covering the defect.

The double pedicle technique is also indicated for radical mastectomy defects with and without irradiation damage to the chest. When using two vascular pedicles for reconstruction of one side of the chest, the abdominal tissue can be transferred as a single flap *(Figs. 10.9, 10.10),* or can be divided in the midline and used as two flaps.

Following a Halsted radical mastectomy, the ipsilateral flap is de-epithelialized and turned over to fill the subclavicular hollow, while the contralateral flap is used to reconstruct the breast wound. If the skin flap is maintained intact, dissection and preservation of the midline fascia are more difficult. Two approaches are recommended. One is to elevate and free the flap from the midline for approximately 3 cm, cutting the fascia 1 cm from the midline on each side. The second approach is to cut the fascia 1 cm from the midline on each side from the deep side. After dividing the deep inferior epigastric vessels and the rectus muscle, the medial aspect of the rectus muscle is bluntly retracted and the fascia is divided from its deep surface and from the midline fascial remnant. The simplest way is to resect the entire fascia, but then mesh would be needed for reconstruction, whereas the surgeon may not be inclined to use it.

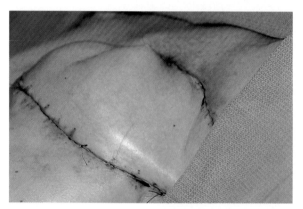

FIG. 10.8

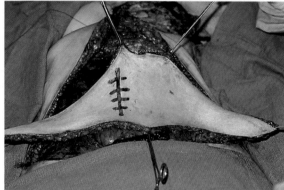

FIG. 10.9

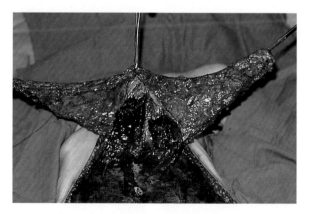

FIG. 10.10

Figures 10.11, 10.12 show the patient 1 month after the TRAM flap with a double pedicle procedure.

Postlumpectomy and Irradiation Defects

A recent area of concern for reconstructive surgeons is the postlumpectomy and irradiation breast deformity. Most difficult to reconstruct, these deformities have to be individualized and assessed carefully. There are no patterns to follow, except that one should avoid local flaps or reshaping the remaining breast tissue. Occasionally, patients are more pleased with the firm and contracted postradiation breast, and an operative procedure is requested for the contralateral normal breast, which more often than not is larger and ptotic.

For patients who present with postradiation persistent and/or recurrent breast carcinoma, total mastectomy is the operation of choice. Reconstruction is essential in these cases, because it brings well-vascularized tissue to the site which ensures satisfactory healing.

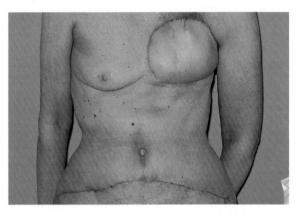

FIG. 10.11

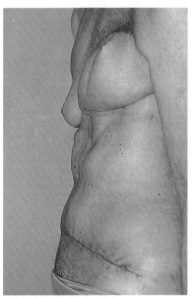

FIG. 10.12

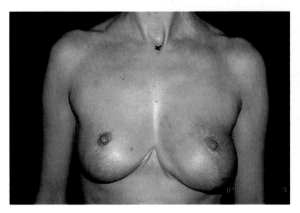

FIG. 10.13

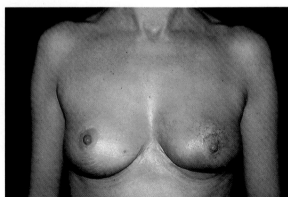

FIG. 10.14

Clinical Cases

Following are cases which demonstrate some of the methods we have used to reconstruct postlumpectomy and postradiation breasts, without recurrence of tumor.

CASE 1. A 49-year-old woman who had mammaplasty 10 years earlier was very concerned about her breast shape *(Fig. 10.13)*. Tumorectomy and irradiation of the left breast 3 years before pre-

sentation had left the breast hard. She requested better shape and symmetry. A careful resection of the lower part of both breasts was accomplished with an eventual recovery *(Fig. 10.14)*.

CASE 2. Tumorectomy irradiation of the left breast of a 50-year-old patient left the breast moderately firm *(Figs. 10.15, 10.16)*. She was treated by mastopexy on the left side and reduction on the right. Results shown are 15 months following the operation *(Figs. 10.17, 10.18)*.

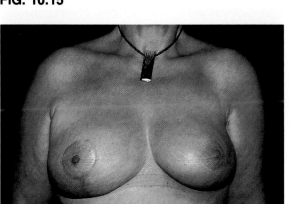

FIG. 10.15

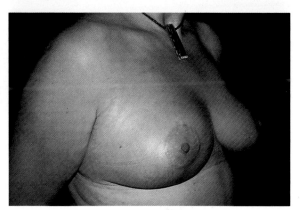

FIG. 10.16

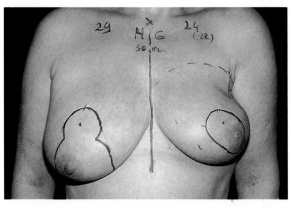

FIG. 10.17

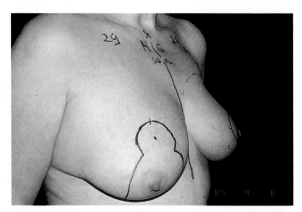

FIG. 10.18

CASES 3 AND 4. A 48-year-old patient, shown 4 years after tumorectomy irradiation, presented with a depression of the upper part of the left breast, which had a normal consistency *(Fig. 10.19)*. Surgery included reduction of the right breast and a latissimus flap without prosthesis on the left side *(Fig. 10.20)*. The result shown is 14 months after the operation *(Fig. 10.21)*.

A similar case occurred in a 47-year-old patient *(Fig. 10.22)*. The latissimus flap was placed in the upper part of the breast to allow repositioning of the nipple and excision of the scar *(Figs. 10.23, 10.24)*.

CASE 5. A 50-year-old patient had tumorectomy irradiation with radionecrosis and recurrence *(Fig. 10.25)*. She was treated with a large excision and bilateral TRAM flap. *Figures 10.26 and 10.27* show the results 5 weeks after the surgical procedure.

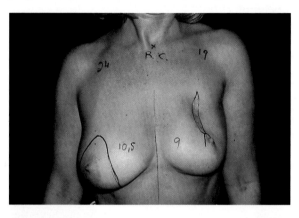

FIG. 10.19

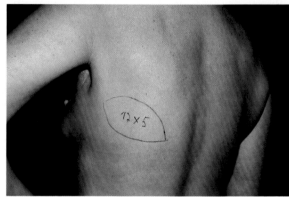

FIG. 10.20

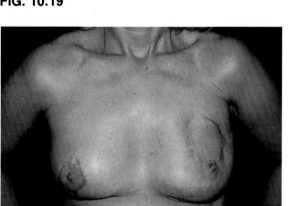

FIG. 10.21

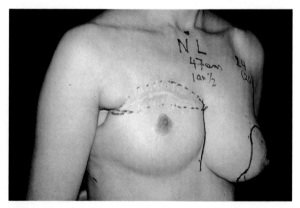

FIG. 10.22

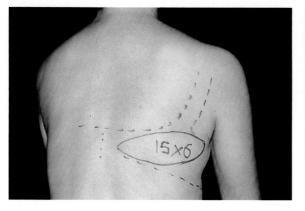

FIG. 10.23

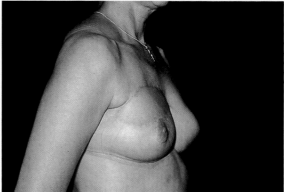

FIG. 10.24

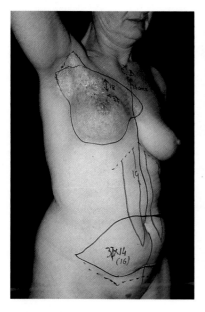

FIG. 10.25

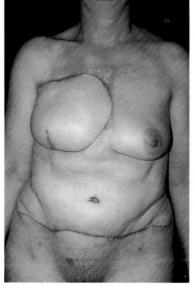

FIG. 10.26

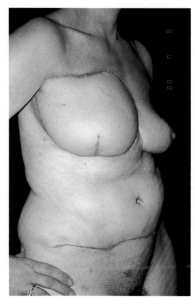

FIG. 10.27

CHAPTER·11

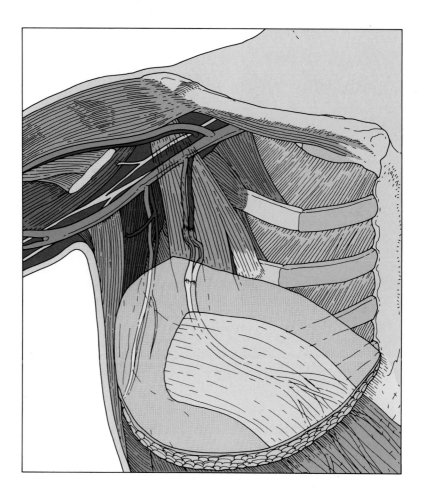

Secondary Breast Reconstruction Alternatives

TRAM FLAP RECONSTRUCTION AFTER IMPLANT COMPLICATIONS

The problems most commonly seen after breast reconstruction with a silicone implant include infection, extrusion of the implant, skin slough of the mastectomy flaps with or without exposure of the prosthesis, and severe fibrous encapsulation with or without intractable pain.

A number of operations have been proposed to correct the resulting deformities in these cases, including open capsulotomies, variations in the type and style of the silicone implants, submuscular placement of the silicone implants, and use of bilateral latissimus dorsi muscle flaps with implants.

Most patients who experience such complications repeatedly demonstrate an intolerance to silicone implants. In such cases, the implants can be

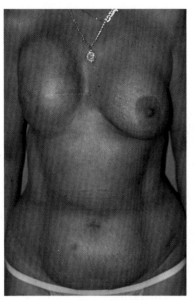

FIG. 11.1

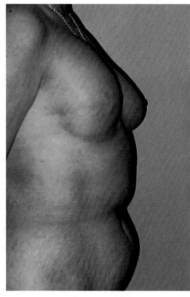

FIG. 11.2

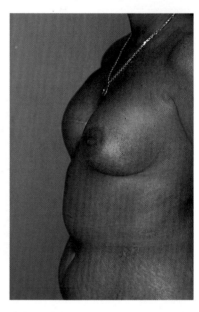

FIG. 11.3

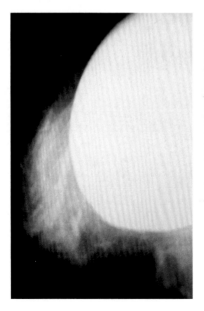

FIG. 11.4

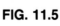

FIG. 11.5

removed and the transverse rectus abdominis muscle (TRAM) flap technique used to reconstruct the breast. In some of these patients, the skin is so scarred and contracted that it is necessary to excise it and replace it. Skin from the lower abdominal flap may be used to provide a good skin covering.

Clinical Case

Figures 11.1–11.3 show a 43-year-old patient who, 8 years previously, underwent bilateral submuscular augmentation mammaplasty. More recently, she developed carcinoma of the right breast and underwent a modified radical mastectomy and immediate staged breast reconstruction by the insertion of a skin expander. The patient is shown after the expander had been inflated with 750 cc of saline. She refused further inflation because of pain, and did not want any modification of her left aug-

mented breast. The option of a TRAM flap reconstruction was presented and accepted.

Figures 11.4 and *11.5* show a normal left mammography that is easy to interpret. The submuscular implant placement disturbs the breast minimally and allows careful monitoring of breast masses.

The skin expander was removed after the transverse mastectomy incision was reopened *(Figs. 11.6, 11.7).* The capsule was opened medially and superiorly, but the inframammary fold was left undisturbed.

The pectoralis major muscle was freed and placed back on the chest wall because the autogenous tissue reconstructive flap goes on top of the pectoralis muscle, under or at the skin level position *(Fig. 11.8).*

As shown in *Figure 11.9,* the contralateral left rectus flap was used. The skin island was outlined from the umbilicus toward the pubis. The entire

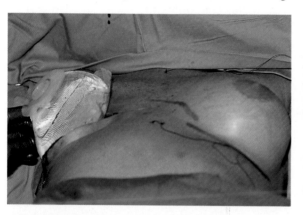

FIG. 11.6

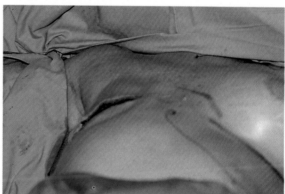

FIG. 11.7

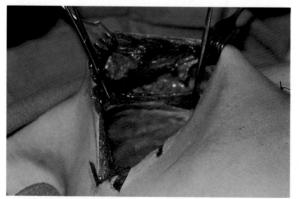

FIG. 11.8

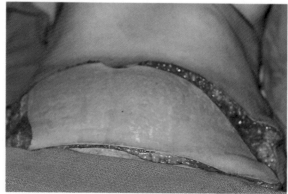

FIG. 11.9

left rectus muscle was elevated with the flap. *Figure 11.10* demonstrates how the flap was passed without difficulty and placed so that the umbilicus was located at approximately 6 o'clock. Zone IV was resected and most of the flap was used.

Figure 11.11 shows the result, a nice breast contour and symmetry with the opposite side. The abdominal wall defect was closed as described in Chapter 4.

Figures 11.12–11.14 illustrate this case 24 months after the TRAM flap reconstruction. The expanded skin and the flap were not sufficient to allow the flap to be de-epithelialized and buried, as was the initial objective. A good portion of added skin was needed to obtain symmetry with the opposite breast.

DE-EPITHELIALIZED TRAM FLAP FOR AUTOGENOUS TISSUE AUGMENTATION

The de-epithelialized TRAM flap is most useful for reconstruction of the breast mound by providing infraclavicular fill while avoiding a skin island on the breast. For this technique to be successful, however, sufficient skin must be available in the breast area to permit adequate projection.

Clinical Case

Figures 11.15 and *11.16* show a 37-year-old patient with a deformity in the left breast after augmentation mammaplasty. The patient had repeatedly demonstrated an intolerance to silicone implants (five unsuccessful operations) and had developed wide and considerable contracture in the submammary area. This caused the nipple to invert and look down. The breast tissue was markedly atrophic from the pressure of the implants. The right breast was large, soft, and had good contour with a 400-cc silicone implant.

To avoid the use of a silicone implant, reconstruction with a de-epithelialized transverse island abdominal flap was planned. The contralateral right rectus abdominis was used. The flap was elevated, taking the entire rectus muscle but leaving a strip of medial and lateral muscle below the umbilicus.

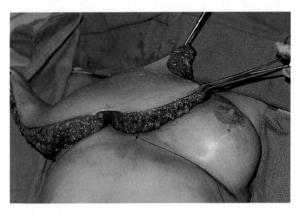

FIG. 11.10

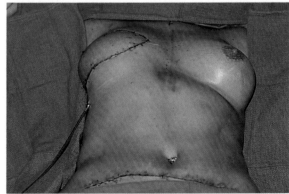

FIG. 11.11

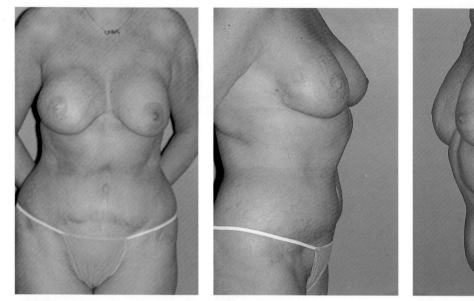

FIG. 11.12   FIG. 11.13   FIG. 11.14

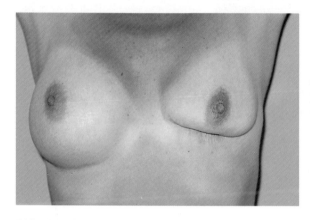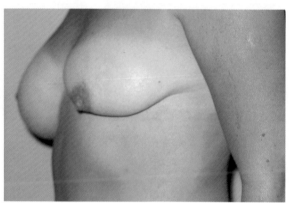

FIG. 11.15   FIG. 11.16

The submammary incision in the left breast was reopened and the inframammary fold was delineated. A tunnel of sufficient size to admit the flap was created from the abdomen to the left breast *(Fig. 11.17)*. Before passing the flap into the chest, the entire flap was de-epithelialized and shaped as a cone to give some projection in the central part. The flap was then tunneled into the chest and placed underneath the previously developed sub-mammary plane and on top of the pectoralis major muscle.

Figures 11.18 and *11.19* show that the de-epithelialized TRAM flap immediately provides a completely natural and permanently soft breast shape. Long-term postoperative photographs are unavailable because the patient declined to return for follow-up, but she indicated being pleased with the result.

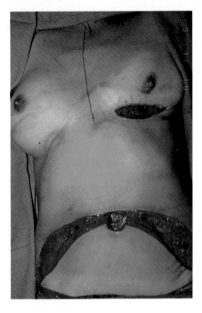

FIG. 11.17

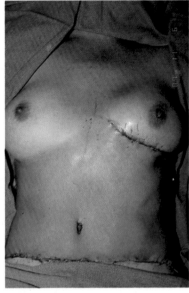

FIG. 11.18

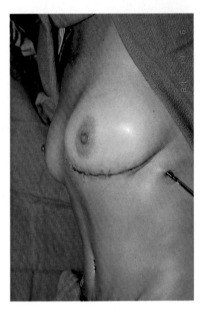

FIG. 11.19

CHAPTER·12

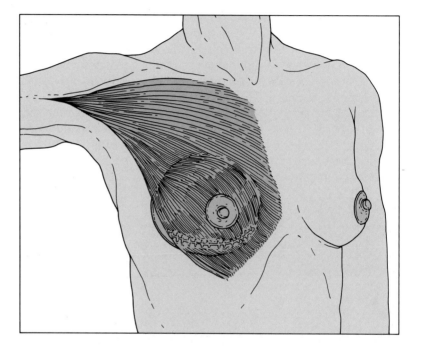

Subcutaneous Mastectomy and Reconstruction

A subcutaneous mastectomy is a resection of the mammary tissue which leaves intact the overlying skin, areola, and nipple. Because the breast is an appendage of the skin, it is almost impossible to remove all the breast tissue. Thus, small amounts of breast tissue are left around the areola, the tail of the breast, or in the subclavicular area. This procedure is usually followed by immediate or delayed implantation of a silicone prosthesis.

The advantage of this procedure is that it usually yields satisfactory cosmetic results. This is particularly true if the skin flaps are dissected beneath the subcutaneous vascular plexus, thus maintaining its blood supply, and if the silicone implants are completely covered with the pectoralis and serratus muscles. Thus, even in instances of superficial necrosis of the skin, the underlying implant does not necessarily have to be removed.

The aesthetic results following subcutaneous mastectomy are better in patients with relatively small, nonptotic breasts. It is less satisfying in pa-

tients with large pendulous breasts. When performing a subcutaneous mastectomy on the contralateral side for prophylaxis in a patient who has already had a modified mastectomy, the results are usually not entirely acceptable because of lack of symmetry. The breast that is reconstructed with a silicone implant on the modified mastectomy side usually has less projection than the one on the subcutaneous side. Sometimes it is preferable to perform a total mastectomy as prophylaxis on the contralateral side using the same type of incision as the modified mastectomy. In this way, the nipple is also removed, both sides are similarly reconstructed, and a bilateral nipple reconstruction is subsequently performed.

The indications for a subcutaneous mastectomy are not entirely clear, but it has been performed on high-risk patients with precancerous mastopathies and on patients with relatively benign conditions, such as cystosarcoma phylloides and giant fibroadenomas, in which most of the breast tissue has

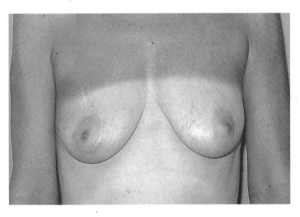

FIG. 12.1

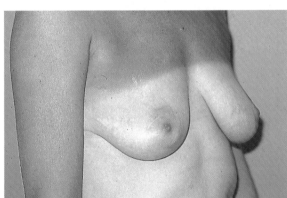

FIG. 12.2

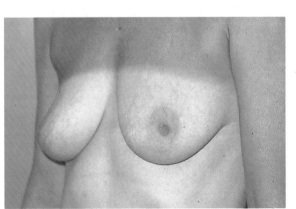

FIG. 12.3

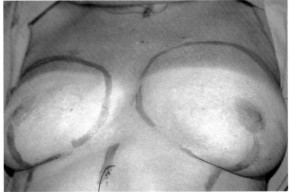

FIG. 12.4

to be removed anyway. It also has been performed on patients with fibrocystic disease, multinodular breasts, and cancerphobia due to a strong family history of breast cancer. It is the operation of choice in gynecomastic males.

Subcutaneous mastectomies are not performed on patients with infiltrating or in situ carcinoma. Subcutaneous mastectomy does not involve excising the skin over and around the tumor, nor does it remove most of the breast tissue. This may explain the relative frequency of recurrences in the residual breast tissue.

Surgical Technique

Figures 12.1–12.3 show a 33-year-old woman who had eight biopsies for fibrocystic disease, all benign. The patient's mother had breast cancer at the age of 50, and her sister developed unilateral breast cancer at the age of 38. Examination of the patient revealed breasts that were pendulous and nodular, with considerable scarring on the right breast from multiple periareolar biopsies. Mammography indicated no significant changes over the previous 2 years.

The objective in subcutaneous mastectomy is to remove most of the breast tissue by freeing it from the overlying skin, subcutaneous tissue, and its attachments along the pectoral fascia. Silicone implants are inserted immediately and are completely covered by the pectoralis and serratus muscles. The skin, while taped superiorly for approximately 10 days to 2 weeks, will shrink and mold around the implant.

Figure 12.4 shows the patient with submammary incisions marked, as well as vertical T-exten-sions at the level of the nipples, which occasionally are used to excise any excess skin—more than can be expected to shrink spontaneously. Note the use of the triangulation principle, in which sutures are placed at the xiphoid and suprasternal notch and used to achieve symmetry.

The extent of the breast tissue begins in the infraclavicular area and extends to almost the parasternal line and toward the axilla to form the axillary tail *(Fig. 12.4)*. An attempt is made to remove most of the breast tissue as marked. The areas of concern are the perforating branches of the internal mammary vessels, parasternally, and the axillary vessels along the axillary tail.

Clinical and anatomic observations have indicated that the breast tissue can be easily freed from the overlying skin if the appropriate plane is found. This plane usually lies at the subcutaneous level; if preserved, the subcutaneous vascular plexus supplies the overlying skin. This plane is relatively easy to find if one uses blunt dissection, which can be started with an empty needle holder *(Fig. 12.5)* and is then expanded with digital dissection by freeing the underlying breast tissue from the overlying subcutaneous tissue and skin. This separates most of the breast tissue attached to the skin in a simple fashion and without any bleeding. This technique is similar to the one used by the cancer surgeon to elevate the somewhat thicker skin flap in an avascular plane, as opposed to the surgeon who elevates a very thin skin flap with considerable bleeding because he is disrupting the subcutaneous plexus and endangering the vascularity of the overlying skin.

Figure 12.6 demonstrates the digital dissection of the underlying breast tissue. An exception to

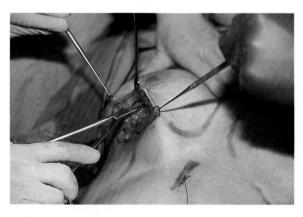

FIG. 12.5

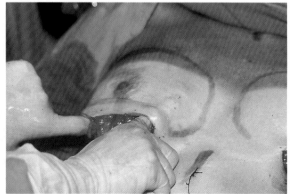

FIG. 12.6

this techniqe is made in areas scarred by previous biopsies and also underneath the nipple itself, where the dissection is done with scissors.

By necessity, a small amount of breast tissue is left underneath the nipple. If there is any question about the breast tissue underneath the nipple, it can be cored out, and the nipple and the areola can be replaced as a free graft. This would, however, negate the advantages of the subcutaneous mastectomy procedure.

Figure 12.7 shows the breast tissue as it is freed from the overlying skin and the pectoralis fascia. As pictured, it is attached to the axillary tail. Using the blunt dissection technique, the surgeon frees the breast tissue from the deep and superficial attachments and avoids the use of sharp instruments that may divide the vessels or the nerves along the anterior axillary line.

Figure 12.8 shows the removed breast specimens that are sent to the pathology laboratory. The specimens may be weighed at this time and replaced with silicone implants of approximately the same volume and weight. This has proven to be helpful, although not an absolutely necessary procedure.

Figure 12.9 shows a 300-cc silicone implant

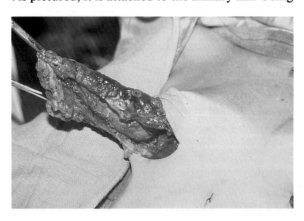

FIG. 12.7

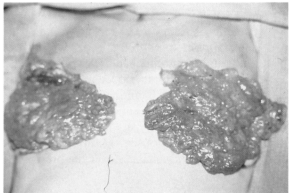

FIG. 12.8

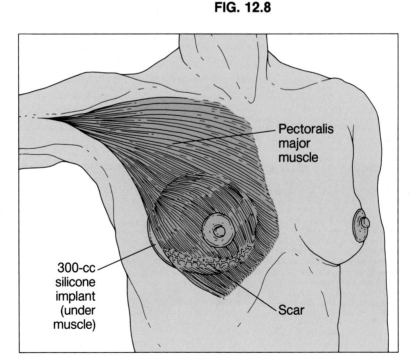

FIG. 12.9

being placed into the opening of the pectoralis major muscle. The surgeon dissects a pocket on the ribs and elevates the anterior rectus sheath, as well as a portion of the serratus muscle. When inserted, the implant is completely protected by the muscle cover. It is essential for the direction and extent of the dissection to be symmetrical on both sides. It must extend just below the inframammary line so that the implant rides relatively low. The ensuing capsular contracture will bring the implant placement higher.

Figure 12.10 shows the submammary incision after it has been closed. A drain should be placed along the anterior axillary line over the muscle, at the subcutaneous level, and brought out through a separate stab wound. This will help the skin mold to the underlying implant. Application of paper tape superiorly allows the skin to shrink.

Figure 12.11 demonstrates a further use of tape. In this case, Microfoam® tape contours the breasts and allows them to mold to the implant. The tape is maintained for approximately 10 days and, if necessary, can be changed and reapplied for a longer period.

Partial skin damage next to the nipple on the left side was noted 1 week after surgery *(Fig. 12.12)*. This was related to the site of previous biopsies. Even if the skin necroses completely, the implant is protected because it is completely covered by muscle.

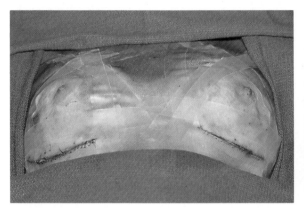

FIG. 12.10

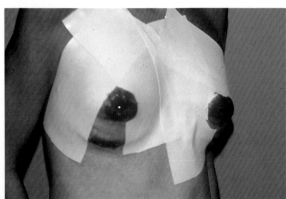

FIG. 12.11

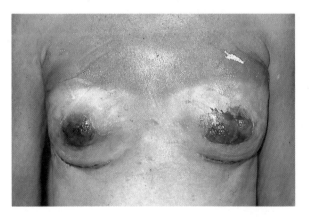

FIG. 12.12

Figures 12.13–12.15 show the patient 3 months after the procedure. The breasts are relatively soft and the cosmetic result is acceptable. The patient still needs to be examined routinely for possible new tumors.

Precautions

Subcutaneous mastectomy has a high rate of complications. These may include skin necrosis, implant exposure, and infection, as well as unsatisfactory aesthetic results due to dimpling of the skin and asymmetry. Consequently, certain precautions should be taken.

The first precaution is the proper choice of pa-tient. A patient with large, pendulous breasts is unlikely to yield a satisfactory result. The same is true of a patient who is obese or requires a unilateral subcutaneous mastectomy because she already has had a modified mastectomy. Obtaining symmetry and acceptable replacement of breast mounds is most difficult on these patients.

The second precaution relates to the technical aspect of skin and subcutaneous tissue dissection. It is of primary importance in this operation that the subcutaneous vascular plexus be preserved. The blunt and finger dissection technique is recommended. These procedures are relatively easy to perform on an unscarred breast, but are more difficult on a breast with previous scarring from bi-

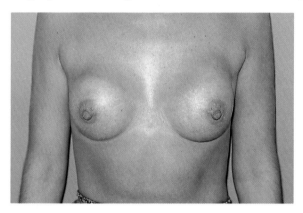

FIG. 12.13

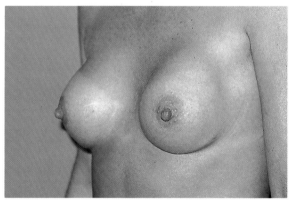

FIG. 12.15

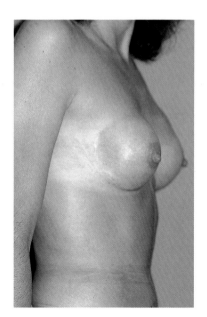

FIG. 12.14

opsies. In scarred areas, precautions must be taken so that, when one resorts to sharp dissection, the overlying dermis is not perforated.

The use of tape to encourage molding and shrinkage of the skin is an excellent principle. The tape should be maintained for 5 days to 3 weeks, depending on the patient's age, amount of extra skin, and amount of striae. As a general rule, younger patients require less taping time because the skin is more elastic.

If the overlying skin has necrosed and there is no evidence of infection, and the implant is completely covered by muscle, one can temporize and treat the overlying skin with topical antibacterials such as Betadine®. This will result in a slow but progressive replacement of the necrotic skin by scar tissue and may prevent the loss of the implant. Betadine does penetrate through the scar and necrotic skin, and prevents the infection from spreading to the deeper planes.

It is a fallacy to think that better symmetry can be obtained by performing a subcutaneous mastectomy on the contralateral side of a patient who has had a modified mastectomy. In such patients, it is preferable to perform a simple mastectomy through a similar incision, removing an ellipse of overlying skin, and reconstructing both breasts similarly. This way their appearance will be symmetrical, with equal projection and equal definition of the inframammary fold.

CHAPTER·13

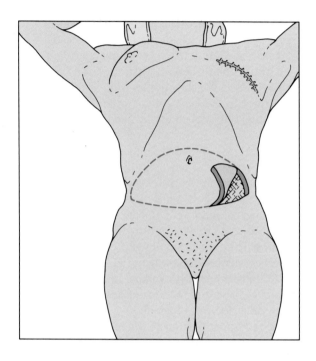

Immediate Breast Reconstruction Using the Free TRAM Flap

James C. Grotting, MD

Advances in microsurgery have paralleled those made in autologous breast reconstruction. The free TRAM flap represents the natural evolution of these developmental concepts as applied to breast reconstruction. The advantages of using this donor site for delayed reconstruction are also applicable in the immediate procedure. At present, the TRAM flap remains the most versatile technique for matching the opposite breast in a single procedure without using implants.

Transferring the TRAM flap as a microsurgical procedure in which the deep inferior epigastric artery and vein are used as the axial pedicle offers several additional advantages. First, the artery is a large-caliber vessel which provides a more reliable inflow to the flap. Second, only a small rectangle of the rectus abdominis muscle needs to be included in the flap, just enough to surround the medial and lateral row of perforating vessels from the deep inferior epigastric pedicle. Taking any muscle below the point where the pedicle meets the muscle is unnecessary. This allows a strip of medial and lateral rectus abdominis muscle to be left intact from the semicircular line to the umbilicus. The lateral strip contains small twigs of intercostal motor nerves which enter along the semilunar line and leave the muscle functionally intact. Above the umbilicus, the entire rectus muscle is left intact and is not dissected from its bed.

Because the upper portion of the rectus abdominis muscle does not need to be dissected for the free TRAM flap transfer, the abdominal skin is undermined only as much as necessary to close the donor defect without tension. No tunneling is required between the abdominal donor site and the mastectomy wound, thereby reducing the excess bleeding that can occur during this portion of the conventional TRAM operation. The epigastric bulge produced by the tunneled rectus muscle, often persistent following surgery using the conventional TRAM flap, is also eliminated. The medial portion of the inframammary fold can be left intact. Therefore, symmetry is improved.

The free TRAM flap is particularly suited for immediate breast reconstruction where the subscapular axis is readily available following axillary dissection. By using the vessels of the subscapular axis as recipient vessels, considerable options are available for folding or molding the flap into a

symmetrical breast. The skin and tissue volume of the mastectomy specimen can be matched more accurately in the context of immediate reconstruction.

Surgical Technique

The patient is positioned supine on an egg crate mattress and warming blanket. We prefer to have the anesthesiologist monitor the patient from the foot of the table using long ventilation tubes. This allows positioning of the microscope and the assistant at the patient's head. A pillow is placed between the knees. The arm on the side of the mastectomy is usually prepped and draped free. Intravenous cannulas are confined to the opposite arm or neck. By warming fluids, gases, and elevating the ambient air temperature, every effort is made to maintain a normal body temperature throughout the procedure. Usually 1 to 2 U of blood is required for this procedure, especially when a simultaneous correction of the opposite breast is performed. Autologous or matched donor blood should be available.

Immediate breast reconstruction using the free TRAM flap is performed using two surgical teams with separate operative instrument sets. If the oncologic surgeon agrees, the mastectomy incisions are planned to spare as much skin of the breast as possible. Usually an incision encompassing the nipple-areola complex and the previous biopsy site, if present, includes a sufficient amount of skin. An oblique extension into the axilla will allow adequate exposure for the axillary dissection and microvascular anastomoses.

The free TRAM flap is designed on the lower abdominal wall in exactly the same manner as the conventional flap, as if one were doing a standard abdominoplasty seeking to keep the scar as low and transverse as possible. The design extends 1 to 2 cm above the umbilicus, with the lower margin running approximately at the level of the suprapubic crease *(Fig. 13.1)*. The contralateral rectus muscle is routinely used. This allows the small segment of rectus muscle to be placed at the point of maximal projection of the newly formed breast and still leave a dependable amount of flap available for filling the infraclavicular hollow and for providing fullness inferiorly and inferolaterally. If chest wall skin must be replaced high in the infra-clavicular area, using the ipsilateral rectus muscle might be a better choice.

The umbilicus is incised circumferentially down to the rectus fascia. The superior incision is bevelled superiorly between the semilunar line on each side to include a few extra periumbilical rec-tus perforators. The ipsilateral side of the flap (with respect to the mastectomy) is raised by 1 to 2 cm beyond the midline. The elevation stops when the medial row of perforators of the contralateral rectus muscle is reached. The fascia is incised at this point. A medial strip of rectus muscle will be left intact *(Fig. 13.2)*.

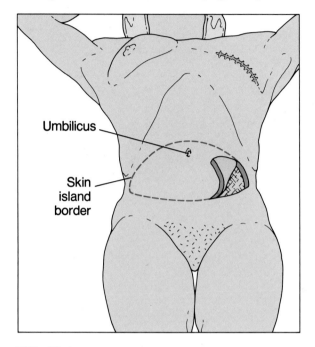

Umbilicus

Skin island border

FIG. 13.1

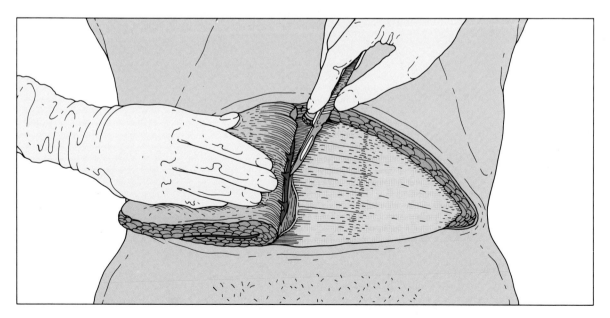

FIG. 13.2

The contralateral side of the flap is then raised until the lateral row of rectus perforators becomes visible. Inferiorly, the flap is raised to the level of the semicircular line, which is commonly marked by a large rectus perforator. At this point, the an-terior rectus sheath is incised forming a rectangle that encompasses the medial, lateral, and most inferior rectus perforators. The intercostal neurovascular bundles are left intact if possible *(Fig. 13.3)*.

The lateral edge of the rectus muscle is then sep-

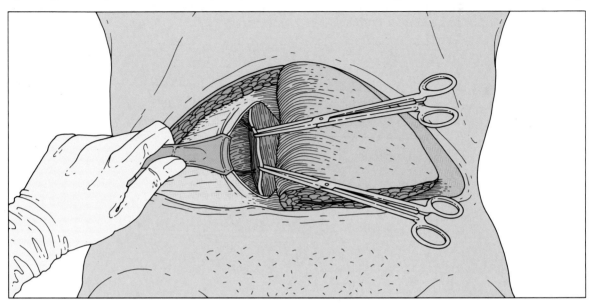

FIG. 13.3

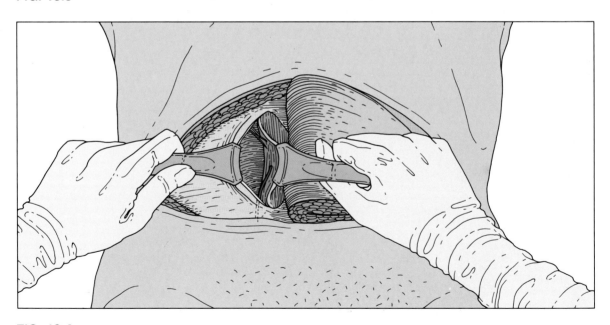

FIG. 13.4

arated just enough so as to identify the entry point of the deep inferior epigastric artery *(Fig. 13.4)*. When this point has been identified, rectus muscle dissection proceeds in rectangular fashion. The muscle is split within its fibers just lateral to this entry point, thereby preserving the lateral row of perforators with the flap. The rectus abdominis muscle can then be divided just inferior to the point where the deep inferior epigastric pedicle meets the muscle. The muscle dissection is then continued medially, again including the medial row of perforators with the flap but preserving an intact medial strip of muscle.

Through this window in the muscle, deep retractors are placed. Using loupe magnification, the deep inferior epigastric artery and two accompanying veins are dissected to their origin from the external iliac vessels through the lateral pelvic wall

(Fig. 13.5). Usually, only two or three small branches are encountered during this dissection, and these are easily controlled using small vessel clips.

In most cases, the amount of time required to raise the flap and complete the mastectomy is similar. Before the superior rectus abdominis muscle is transected, the recipient vessels must be explored to determine their adequacy for microvascular anastomosis. The subscapular axis can be examined following completion of the mastectomy to identify the recipient vessels that are best matched by size to the inferior epigastric pedicle. We prefer using the thoracodorsal artery and vein proximal to the serratus branch for end-to-end anastomosis. We believe this provides the most reliable inflow with good match of vessel caliber, as well as more flexibility for placing the flap in the

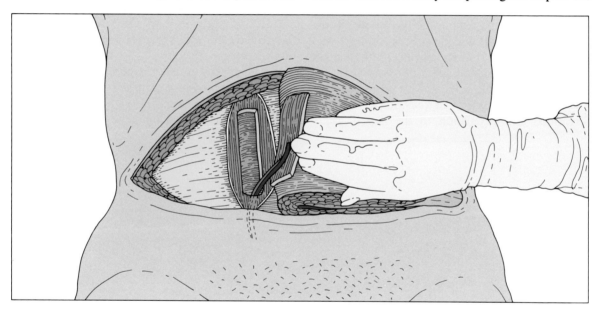

FIG. 13.5

proper position *(Fig. 13.6)*. Also, axial flow to the latissimus dorsi muscle is maintained by retrograde flow through the serratus branch if this muscle were ever required for secondary coverage.

After adequate inflow has been established, the central remaining portion of the rectus abdominis muscle is divided superiorly so that the entire flap is allowed to perfuse only on the deep inferior epigastric artery and accompanying veins. Until this point, the flap could still be transferred as a conventional TRAM if either donor or recipient vessels were considered inadequate. With warming, the circulation of the flap appears to stabilize, and after 10 to 15 minutes the flap can be transferred.

The deep inferior epigastric pedicle is then divided at its origin through the lateral pelvic wall, and the flap is safely transferred to the mastectomy site. The flap can either be positioned on the upper arm allowing the vessels to fall into the axillary wound, or it can be temporarily positioned in the mastectomy wound and the vessels brought into the axillary defect. It often helps to tilt the patient toward the contralateral side to improve the visibility into the axilla.

End-to-end microvascular anastomoses are then performed and circulation to the flap is estab-lished. A drain is placed in the axilla, and the latissimus muscle is sutured to the serratus to partially close the axilla. The axillary skin flap then can also be sutured to close the axilla and help recreate the lateral and inferolateral aspect of the breast and inframammary fold. The small segment of rectus muscle is sutured to the pectoralis major muscle at the point where maximum projection of the breast is desired *(Fig. 13.7)*. Care is taken to observe the vessels during this maneuver to ensure that they are under no tension. The flap can then be rotated and folded to replace the tissues removed with the mastectomy specimen. If abundant breast skin is available, most of the flap can be de-epithelialized and only a small monitoring disc of skin be left at the anticipated position of the nipple-areola complex. If necessary, the entire flap can often be safely used, as zone IV frequently receives adequate perfusion. In our experience, however, it has rarely been necessary to use the entire flap to have enough tissue for symmetry with the opposite side.

If a large skin excision is necessary for an adequate mastectomy, it is helpful to make a template of the shape of the skin excision before incising the mastectomy flaps. This template can then be used

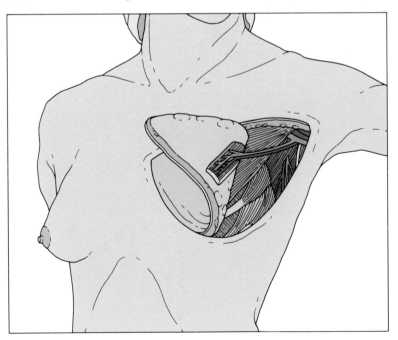

FIG. 13.6

as a guide for locating the mastectomy flaps over the de-epithelialized TRAM flap. A second drain is usually left beneath the flap.

If a reduction or mastopexy on the opposite side is desirable, we prefer to do this before molding the TRAM flap. We have found that it is easier to mold the TRAM flap to match the corrected opposite breast rather than to perform the opposite correction in a second operation. It is best to have a second team perform the opposite breast correction while the mastectomy is being done or while the TRAM flap is being raised.

The closure of the abdominal wall is considerably less difficult than with the conventional TRAM procedure. The anterior rectus sheath and medial and lateral strips of rectus muscle are easily reapproximated with O prolene sutures. The umbilicus may be pulled over during this closure, but this usually can be easily corrected by imbricating the fascia on the opposite side. The entire reconstruction is improved if formal abdominoplasty techniques are used for the abdominal wall closure. This may include using bilateral external oblique advancement flaps. The superior abdominal skin and subcutaneous tissue are undermined as much as necessary to allow closure of the flap

donor site without tension. The umbilicus is sutured to the deep fascia and brought through in an appropriate position. The area around the new umbilicus is defatted to recreate the periumbilical depression. Two large suction drains are placed on each side, and the wound is closed.

Molding of the breast is best accomplished with the patient in the sitting position so that symmetry can be examined. The time spent carefully molding the breast in the initial operation reduces the likelihood of corrective revisions. Nipple and areola reconstruction is always performed 3 months later—unless chemotherapy has been initiated, in which case reconstruction is usually delayed until the completion of chemotherapy.

Postoperative Management

The patient is transferred directly to a hospital bed with her head elevated 20 to 30° and the knees elevated, supported, and flexed. The patient is asked to maintain her shoulder on the side of the reconstruction between 30 and 90° of abduction to avoid compression or stretching of the microvascular anastomoses. This positioning is continued for approximately 10 days.

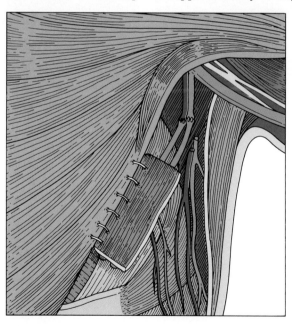

FIG. 13.7

With the exception of a single aspirin tablet daily starting in the postoperative period, no other anticoagulants are used. Fluids are administered intravenously to maintain the urine volume at approximately 1 cc/kg/hr. Ideally, the hematocrit should be kept around 30.

The patient is allowed out of bed on the first postoperative day, with assistance. She is encouraged to walk when she feels able. Feeding is resumed when bowel tones appear and the patient feels hungry. We customarily use perioperative antibiotics, but feel that this is optional.

Drains are removed as flow diminishes to less than 30 cc/day. Keeping the patient hospitalized merely because drains are in is unnecessary. Most patients go home between the fifth and seventh postoperative day.

Prior to discharge, the patient is fitted with a soft

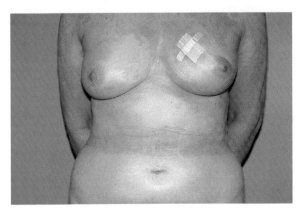

FIG. 13.8

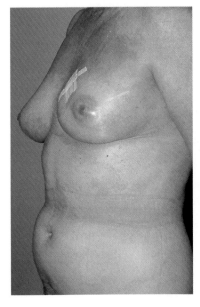

FIG. 13.9

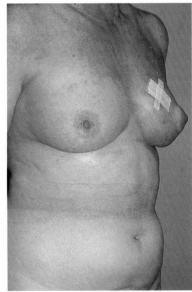

FIG. 13.10

brassiere to help support and mold the breast, as well as to define the inframammary fold. Care is taken to avoid any axillary compression which might damage the vascular pedicle.

Clinical Case

Figures 13.8–13.10 show a 54-year-old patient with carcinoma of the left breast. She underwent a left modified radical mastectomy and immediate left breast reconstruction using an ipsilateral free microvascular TRAM flap. The end-to-end anastomoses were performed between the deep inferior epigastric artery and the thoracodorsal artery. The thoracodorsal veins were then anastomosed to the inferior epigastric veins in similar fashion. The segment of the rectus muscle was then attached to the edge of the pectoralis major muscle.

Figures 13.11–13.13 show satisfactory results 8 months after reconstruction. The nipple-areola complex was reconstructed at 3 months under local anesthesia.

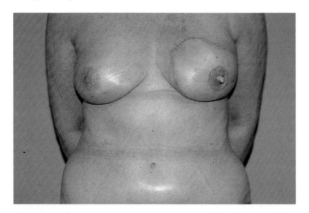

FIG. 13.11

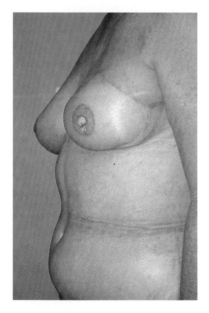

FIG. 13.12

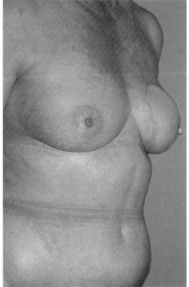

FIG. 13.13

CHAPTER·14

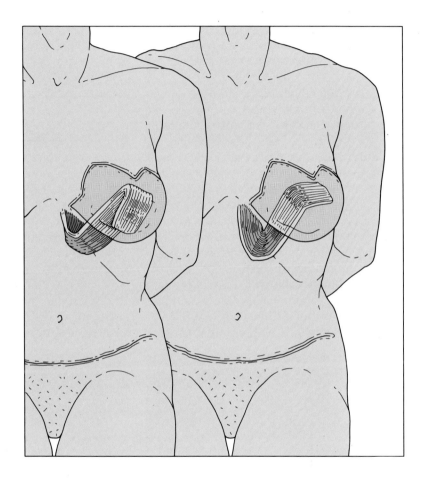

Complications

RECURRENT CARCINOMA IN THE RECONSTRUCTED BREAST

Persistent and/or recurrent carcinoma in the reconstructed breast is always a possibility. As more and more immediate reconstructions of the breast are performed, the expected normal rate of local recurrences in any mastectomy is 3 to 5%.

Most recurrences occur at the subcutaneous level. The fear of hiding the recurrence under a flap has not been warranted. If there is bony recurrence, it will manifest by pain, and radiograms and bone scans will confirm the presence of metastasis.

Making the differential diagnosis between the rare (but possible) recurrent tumor around the scar or in the subcutaneous tissues, and the more commonly occurring fat necrosis in the transverse island abdominal flap presents a challenge. Clinical observation indicates that fat necrosis usually is apparent from the early postoperative course (2 to 3 weeks), and that it persists. The indurated area is not tender, nor does it drain. The recurrent tumor may appear months after the reconstruction. The site is relatively flat and usually increases in size.

Diagnosis to distinguish between fat necrosis and recurring tumor begins with xeroradiography or mammography. Mammograms are usually not indicated on reconstructed breasts with a TRAM flap. The next step is fine needle aspiration. If it shows fat necrosis, the patient is followed and advised. If, on the other hand, aspiration shows tumor cells, an open excisional biopsy is performed.

The treatments of recurring cancer vary. Most of our patients who have presented with recurrent carcinoma in the scar have been treated by radiotherapy with or without additional chemotherapy. Most patients are likely to have already received chemotherapy. The success rate is not very satisfactory, particularly with radiotherapy. The option of removing the reconstructed breast, however painful a decision, should be considered. In every case, an excisional biopsy with adequate tumor margins is performed.

Clinical Case

Figure 14.1 shows a patient 1 year after mastectomy for carcinoma of the left breast. Because the right breast had been previously augmented, an effort was made in the reconstruction to match the opposite side. *Figure 14.2* shows the patient 7 months following reconstruction.

Nine months after reconstruction, the patient presented with a palpable indurated mass at approximately 12 o'clock *(Fig. 14.3)*. Following needle aspiration, the excisional biopsy confirmed carcinoma of the breast. The tumor persisted and was treated with radiation of a very high dose, in-

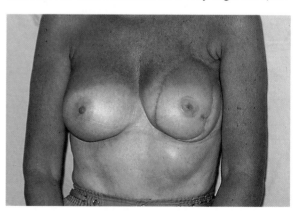

FIG. 14.2

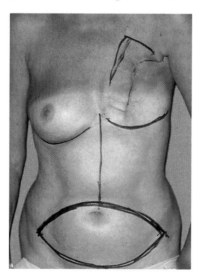

FIG. 14.1

cluding hyperthermic radiotherapy. This treatment did not shrink the mass *(Fig. 14.4)*. The patient also received chemotherapy, but died 15 months after reconstruction.

PARTIAL FLAP NECROSIS—FLAP EXTENDED BEYOND THE LOWER MIDLINE ABDOMINAL SCAR

Extending a flap beyond a lower midline abdominal scar gives unreliable results. Although there are reports of survival of the flap beyond the scar, necrosis of the tissue lying past the scar is more likely to occur. If more hemiabdominal tissue is needed for reconstruction, the use of bilateral rectus abdominis muscles as carriers is advised.

Clinical Case

Figure 14.5 shows a thin patient who was to undergo reconstruction with a transverse island abdominal flap following right mastectomy. A lower midline scar was present, and the flap was based on the left rectus abdominis muscle. At the same time the patient underwent a left subcutaneous mastectomy.

The area of necrosis extended just beyond the area of the scar and there was also partial necrosis of the nipple on the left side *(Fig. 14.6)*. Impending necrosis of flaps or frank necrosis is treated by frequent applications of Betadine® ointment, which penetrates the scar or the underperfused tissue, prevents infection, and results in demarcation of the necrotic tissue. Once the area of tissue loss

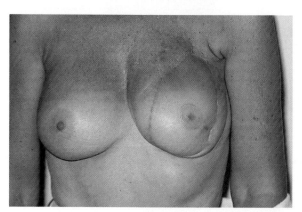

FIG. 14.3

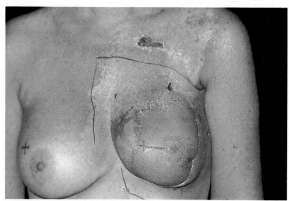

FIG. 14.4

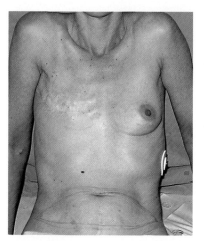

FIG. 14.5

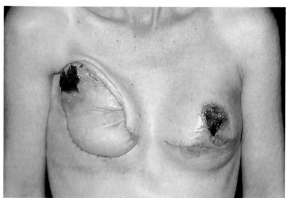

FIG. 14.6

has been defined, it is removed and the wound is allowed to heal by contracture or is closed with a split skin graft *(Fig. 14.7)*.

COMPLEX RECONSTRUCTION FOR SILICONE INJECTIONS OF THE BREAST

The number of patients who have undergone injections of silicone for breast augmentation is not known, nor is the percentage of patients who have complications following silicone injections.

In such cases, as much silicone as possible should be removed, and reconstruction of the breast may or may not be necessary. The second option is to perform a staged resection of the silicone with reconstruction of the breast by a variety of methods.

When silicone is injected into the tissues, it usually diffuses widely throughout them and a pseudocapsule is formed around it. Silicone can migrate over long distances, usually following tissue planes. It may also be picked up by the regional

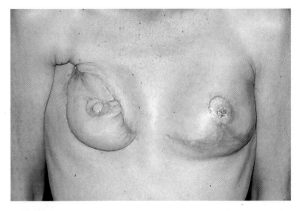

FIG. 14.7

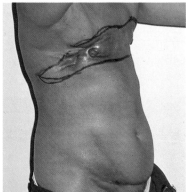

FIG. 14.8

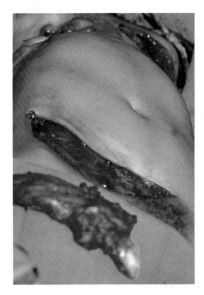

FIG. 14.9

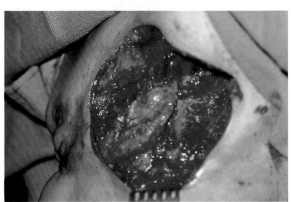

FIG. 14.10

lymph nodes. Other than the rare case of "adjuvant type disease," there are no other known systemic effects.

Clinical Cases

CASE 1. The patient was a 45-year-old Oriental woman who underwent silicone injections for breast augmentation 10 years earlier *(Fig. 14.8)*. A considerable amount of silicone had migrated into the chest, the inguinal regions, and was present throughout the abdomen. The silicone was removed from the chest alongside an ellipse of skin, and from the inguinal regions through a suprapubic incision *(Fig. 14.9)*.

Figure 14.10 shows the silicone which adhered close to the underlying ribs. The removed silicone was contained in a pseudocapsule *(Fig. 14.11)*. Because of the migration of the silicone throughout the tissues, its complete removal was impossible. The larger pieces that were easily palpable were removed.

Healing was satisfactory. Reconstruction of the breast was not offered to the patient, because the persistent amount of silicone in the chest and abdominal walls could present problems in the future.

CASE 2. A 48-year-old woman had undergone silicone injections for breast augmentation 20 years earlier. Her problems began to develop 15 years following the injections. Areas of localized inflammation were treated by partial removal of the extruding silicone.

Figures 14.12–14.14 show the preoperative status. Destruction of the chest wall from multiple scars as well as palpable silicone throughout the chest, particularly along the parasternal and left in-

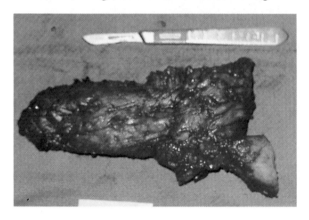

FIG. 14.11

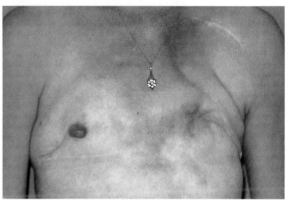

FIG. 14.12

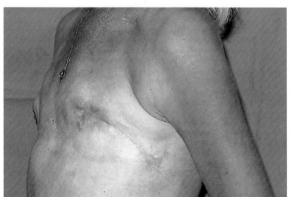

FIG. 14.13

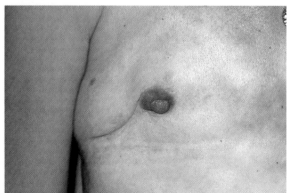

FIG. 14.14

fraclavicular areas, are apparent. Despite the multiple incisions, there was no evidence of localized inflammation or infection at the time.

A staged removal of the silicone, as well as reconstruction of the breasts were carried out. A portion of skin and as much of the silicone as possible were removed from the chest wall through a transverse incision in the right chest.

Following satisfactory healing, a right latissimus dorsi myocutaneous unit was transposed to the chest for reconstruction of the breast. The skin island was placed in the inframammary region, disregarding the previous transverse scar. For adequate projection, a saline inflatable implant was inserted at the same time *(Fig. 14.15).*

In another operation, a considerable portion of the silicone was resected from the lower aspect of the left chest, as well as a considerable portion from the subclavicular area. A rather large defect was closed with a transverse island abdominal flap (outlined and elevated in *Fig. 14.16,* transposed in *Fig. 14.17*).

A large concavity remained in the left subclavicular area following the removal of the silicone which had invaded the underlying pectoralis major muscle. The deformity simulated that seen in a Halsted-type radical mastectomy. To fill this concavity, a de-epithelialized island latissimus dorsi myocutaneous flap was transposed to the subclavicular region. The L-shaped pattern of the

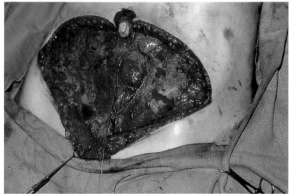

FIG. 14.16

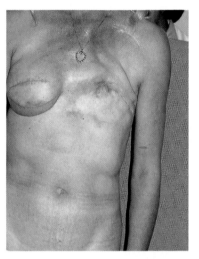

FIG. 14.15

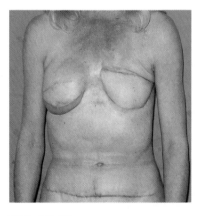

FIG. 14.17

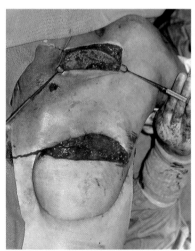

FIG. 14.18

concavity involved the subclavicular area and extended along the left parasternal area. This pattern was transferred to the back, where the skin island was outlined, de-epithelialized, and transposed *(Fig. 14.18)*. The transposed unit was sutured to the clavicle and buried under the skin *(Fig. 14.19)*.

Figure 14.20 shows the patient with healed latissimus dorsi scars, which are mirror images. *Figure 14.21* shows the patient following nipple reconstruction as well as the insertion of a small saline implant on the left side.

Other options are available for treating silicone injection complications. Bilateral transverse island abdominal flaps may be used to resurface the chest walls, with or without saline implants to provide added projection. Use of the de-epithelialized latissimus dorsi skin island for filling the subclavicular area is an option. The latissimus dorsi muscle alone, even if it is folded on itself, does not provide satisfactory filling of that area. The muscle usually atrophies and the concavity persists. On the other hand, the added fullness of the de-epithelialized skin island does give lasting correction of the subclavicular concavity.

EXPOSURE OF THE IMPLANT IN POLAND'S SYNDROME

Poland's syndrome presents itself in different degrees of severity. In every case, there is an abnormality of the chest wall and of the breast which is much more apparent in the female.

The simplest way to treat Poland's syndrome in women has been with the insertion of an appropriate silicone implant in an effort to match the opposite side. The use of an expander-type implant should be considered if the treatment is begun at puberty, before the patient is fully grown, so that saline can be injected to match the development of the opposite breast.

In most female patients with Poland's syndrome, the involved breast is usually smaller than

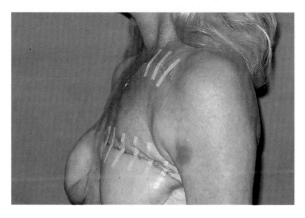

FIG. 14.19

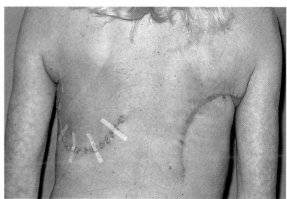

FIG. 14.20

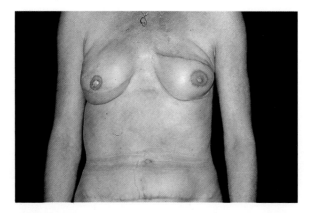

FIG. 14.21

the contralateral one, and the inframammary fold is higher. The nipple also is smaller and higher, and there is a variable concavity in the upper chest depending on the partial or complete absence of the pectoralis major muscle. There is loss of the anterior axillary fold, but the posterior axillary fold is usually present.

The following observations are based on a limited experience of treating patients with Poland's syndrome with silicone implants.

1. It is difficult to find a clear-cut submammary plane, particularly if the patient is at puberty and is moderately obese. Breast and fat are difficult to differentiate. Because there is no pectoralis major muscle, one could mistakenly dissect at the serratus plane.
2. The dissection to create an adequate pocket is quite difficult.
3. Because the involved breast is usually smaller and the inframammary fold higher,

the implant should be placed lower. Dissecting below the incision is necessary.
4. Exposure of the breast implant is not unusual *(Fig. 14.25)*. When it occurs, it is best to remove the implant. At least 6 months should elapse before reinsertion, at which time an expander-type implant is used and is expanded slowly.

Clinical Case

Figures 14.22 and 14.23 show a patient with Poland's syndrome in the preoperative state. An exposed implant required removal 2 weeks after surgery *(Fig. 14.24)*.

ABDOMINAL HERNIA

An abdominal hernia, or pseudohernia, following a TRAM flap is due to a disruption of the vertical fascial closure or to a failure to approximate the

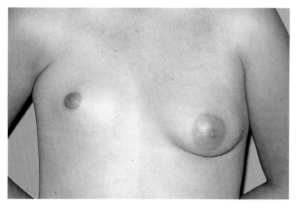

FIG. 14.22

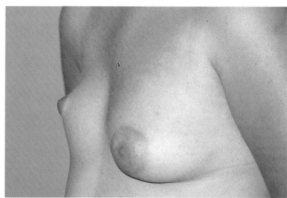

FIG. 14.23

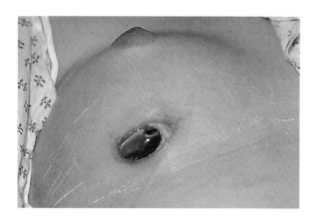

FIG. 14.24

internal oblique layer below the semicircular line. Closure of this defect must be technically perfect to avoid postoperative disruption and can be avoided if the following operative guidelines are observed.

The components of the abdominal wall below the semicircular line must be preserved, including the pyramidal muscle, the anterior rectus sheath, and the distal end of the rectus muscles. This step is most important, since below this level the principal structural support is concentrated in the anterior rectus sheath, whereas the posterior sheath is composed only of the thin fascia transversalis.

Hartrampf[2] also recommends preserving the medial and lateral third of the rectus and its fascia. This decreases the tension necessary for closure of the vertical gap in the abdominal wall. It should be emphasized that two vertical ligamentous structures must be spared: the linea alba and as much lateral fascia as possible, medial to the linea semilunaris. This latter structure offers a solid anchorage for the midline suture of the lateral muscles or synthetic mesh in either a unilateral or bilateral closure.

The anterior rectus sheath comprises the junction of the external oblique and the anterior layer of the internal oblique. The two layers are fused above the umbilicus, but are separate and distinct below the umbilicus. This deep aponeurotic layer composed of the internal oblique, and even the

transversus, has a strong tendency to retract laterally and can be easily missed during closure of the donor area. Such a defect would lack the support of the strongest layer, and postoperative bulging would probably occur *(Figs. 14.25, 14.26).*[1] A careful approximation of both aponeurotic sheets must be secured.

Imbrication of the internal oblique muscle over the external border of the rectus sheaths and mobilization of the external oblique aponeuroses (as shown in Chapter 4) has the obvious advantage of tightening the abdomen and repositioning the umbilicus.[3] This may account for the improvement obtained in total reshaping of the abdomen. Of note, in the past 4 years we have not had a postoperative hernia, which explains the absence of an illustrative case.

A DOUBLE FOLD OF THE VASCULAR PEDICLE OF THE TRAM FLAP

When raising, rotating, and shaping the TRAM flap, special attention should be given to the location of the vascular pedicle. The new breast flap will not tolerate double folding or excessive twisting of the pedicle. The flap becomes blue and immediate reexploration is indicated. The following clinical case illustrates this complication and shows how it was corrected by immediate reexploration.

FIG. 14.25

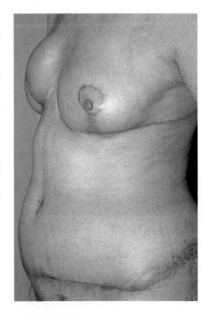

FIG. 14.26

Clinical Case

The patient, a 41-year-old white woman, had a left modified radical mastectomy, chemotherapy, and radiation therapy for breast carcinoma with positive lymph nodes 4 years before presentation.

Figures 14.27 and 14.28 show the patient following a prophylactic right simple mastectomy and reconstruction with bilateral TRAM flaps. In the immediate postoperative period, the left flap appeared to be mottled and venous obstruction was suspected. Reexploration was indicated 3 hours postoperatively.

After removal of the sutures, it was noticed that the vascular pedicle of the rectus muscle had a double fold that was obstructing the venous return (Figs. 14.29, 14.30). The double fold was corrected and the flap reset, with the flap folded in a 90° turn as opposed to a double fold (Fig. 14.31). Good color returned to the flap, and the postoperative course was uncomplicated (Fig. 14.32).

CONVENTIONAL TRAM FLAP WITH MICROVASCULAR ENHANCEMENT

The viability of the flap depends on the adequate vascular supply to the tissues entering through the superior epigastric vessels. If the flap is mottled

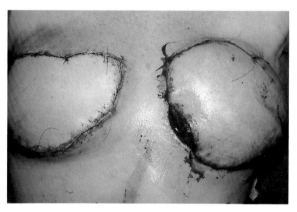

FIG. 14.27

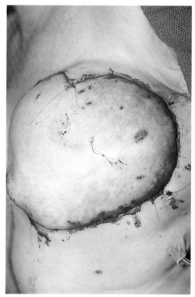

FIG. 14.28

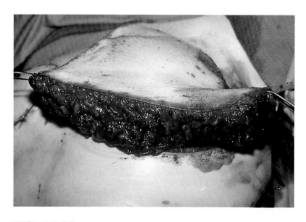

FIG. 14.29

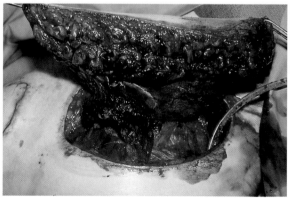

FIG. 14.30

and cold, there is no visible improvement after releasing some of the sutures, and a hematoma is not present, immediate reexploration is indicated, including inspection of the superior epigastric vessels. It is not unusual to find distention of the veins with a functioning artery. If the mottled appearance of the flap does not improve while the flap is free of sutures and untwisted, the surgeon should be prepared to augment the flow by microvascular hookup of the deep inferior epigastric vessels to an appropriate recipient in the axilla, usually the thoracodorsal vessels.

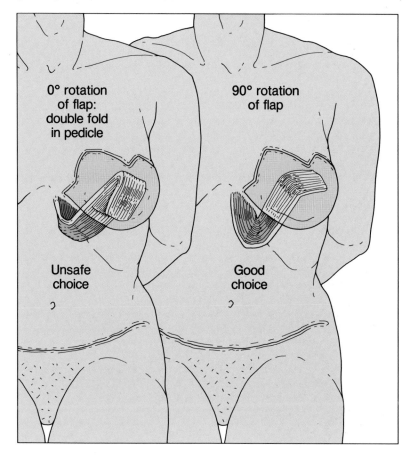

FIG. 14.31

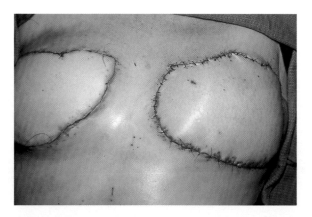

FIG. 14.32

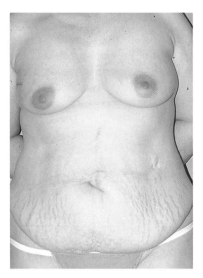

FIG. 14.33

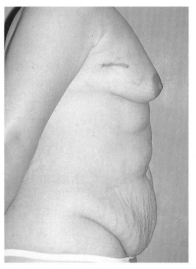

FIG. 14.34

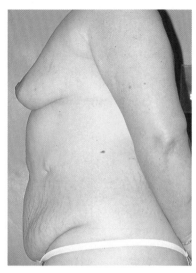

FIG. 14.35

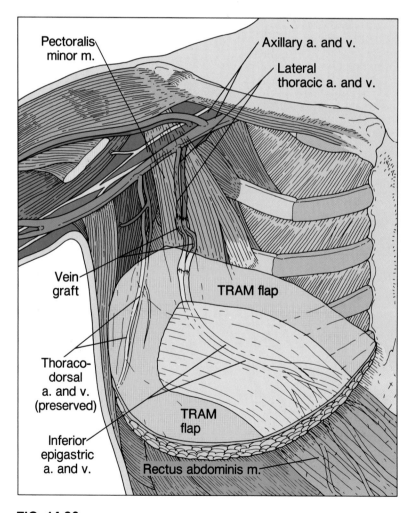

FIG. 14.36

COMPLICATIONS

Clinical Case

A 34-year-old woman had undergone radiation therapy for Hodgkin's disease 12 years earlier *(Figs. 14.33–14.35)*. Radiation portals included the neck, the mediastinum, and a portion of her right breast. She developed secondary hypothyroidism. Her abdomen was moderately obese, with an apron hanging over the pubis, and displayed considerable striae and a left paramedian scar. The patient developed carcinoma of the right breast, and a modified radical mastectomy was performed with immediate breast reconstruction using the transverse abdominal island flap pedicled on the contralateral rectus abdominis muscle.

Because in the immediate postoperative period the flap appeared to be affected by venous congestion, reexploration was indicated. The TRAM flap had good arterial flow through the superior epigastric artery, and distention of the epigastric vein was observed. The inflow and outflow were improved with microvascular vein grafting of the inferior epigastric artery and vein to the serratus branch artery and vein in the right axilla *(Fig. 14.36)*. The abdominal incision was not reopened *(Fig. 14.37)*. The TRAM flap improved substantially in color, and healed satisfactorily.

Using the serratus vascular pedicle and maintaining the thoracodorsal artery and vein intact permits the latissimus dorsi flap to be used later, if

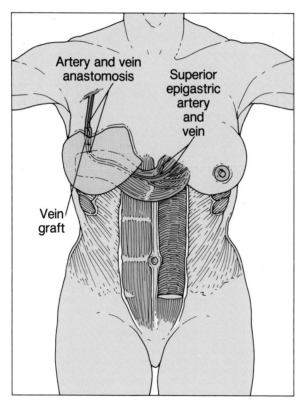

FIG. 14.37

needed. The reconstructed right breast showed a satisfactory result, as seen 2 weeks postoperatively *(Figs. 14.38–14.40)*.

EARLY ABDOMINAL REEXPLORATION

Distension and rigidity of the abdominal wall after TRAM flap reconstruction can simulate an acute abdominal catastrophe even in the absence of per-

forated viscus. Aggravating circumstances that can confuse the correct diagnosis, such as chronic constipation, use of narcotics, imbalance of electrolytes, and hypokalemia must always be kept in mind. After consultation with the general surgeon, a decision usually is made to open the abdomen through a midline incision rather than to reopen the suprapubic incision. This permits exposure of the underlying fascial closure and adequate explo-

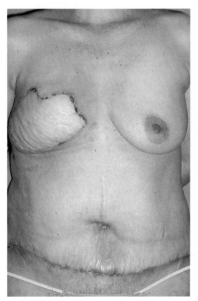

FIG. 14.38

FIG. 14.39

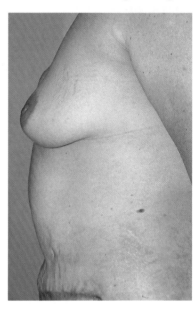

FIG. 14.40

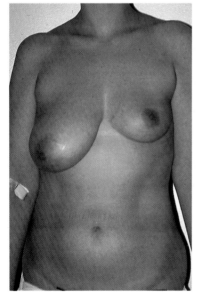

FIG. 14.41

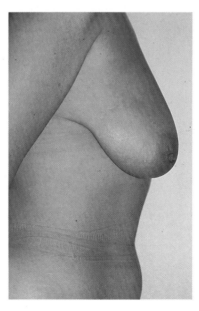

FIG. 14.42

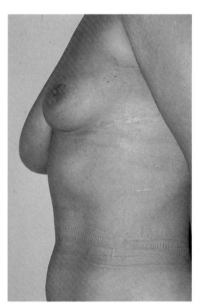

FIG. 14.43

COMPLICATIONS

ration of the abdomen. Postexploratory abdominal closure is not difficult, but, if it cannot be secured, a prosthetic mesh overlay should be applied.

Clinical Case

A 37-year-old white female with carcinoma of the left breast had a past medical history remarkable for Ewing's sarcoma of the left lower extremity for which, at the age of 14, she received high radiation therapy to the leg *(Figs. 14.41–14.43)*. She was subsequently diagnosed as having pulmonary metastasis to the left lung and received extensive radiation to the left lung through both anterior and posterior ports. The tumor did not respond to radiation, and she subsequently underwent a thoracotomy and a partial pulmonary resection that included removal of the tumor mass.

The patient was left with residual moderate scoliosis of the thoracic vertebras, as well as a left breast which was hyperpigmented and substantially smaller than the right breast. She developed breast carcinoma in the left breast as a result of the carcinogenic effect of irradiation. The latency period was approximately 23 years. The patient was obviously not a candidate for breast conservation with radiation because of her prior radiation to the left breast.

She underwent a right total mastectomy and left total mastectomy with lower axillary lymph node dissection. Immediate breast reconstruction with bilateral TRAM flaps was performed. Standard closure of the abdominal wall was performed without difficulty. Prosthetic mesh was not used.

Five weeks after surgery the patient began experiencing intermittent bloating and developed acute midabdominal pain, principally located on the left side. On physical examination, the abdomen appeared rigid, tense, and tympanitic, and had exquisite and diffuse tenderness. The abdominal flat plate shown in *Figure 14.44* revealed a large amount of air collected in the upper portion of the abdomen suggesting a perforated viscus. Exploratory laparotomy was indicated. *Figure 14.45* shows massive dilatation of the left colon with possible volvulus and adhesions. The colon was decompressed and lysis of adhesions was performed. No perforated viscus was found. Postoperatively, a superficial infection was detected in the wound.

REFERENCES

1. Drever JM, Hodson-Walker N: Closure of the donor defect for breast reconstruction with rectus abdominis myocutaneous flaps. *Plast Reconstr Surg* 1985; 76:558.
2. Hartrampf CR Jr: Abdominal wall competence in transverse abdominal island flap operations. *Ann Plast Surg* 1984; 12:139.
3. Psillakis JM: Plastic surgery of the abdomen with improvement in the body contour. *Clin Plast Surg* 1984; 2:465.

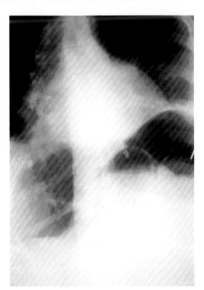

FIG. 14.44

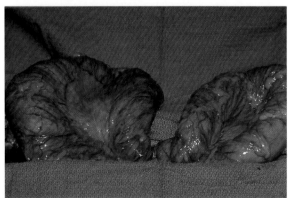

FIG. 14.45

CHAPTER·15

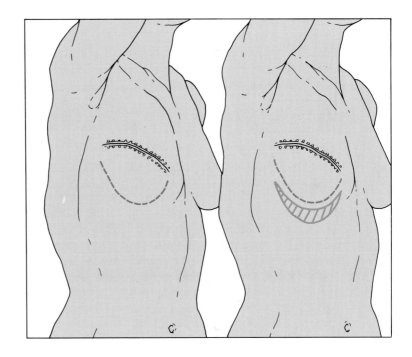

Postmastectomy Reconstruction with Ipsilateral Upper Rectus Myocutaneous Flap

Rama P. Mukherjee, MD

Depending on the availability of local tissue, several methods may be used for breast reconstruction. Breasts can be rebuilt with submuscular silicone implants or with tissue expanders followed by replacement with permanent silicone implants. When adequate local tissue is not available due to surgery or radiotherapeutic damage, distant tissue is needed in the form of myocutaneous pedicle or free flaps, such as a latissimus dorsi or rectus abdominis myocutaneous flap. Gluteal flaps also have been used as free flaps to reconstruct breasts, with excellent results. Currently, the most popular method includes reconstruction with rectus abdominis myocutaneous flaps. The use of the upper rectus flaps will be discussed here.[6]

Anatomic Considerations

The rectus abdominis muscle originates at the pubic crest and pubic ligament, and inserts over the costal cartilages of the fifth, sixth, and seventh ribs. It is situated on each side of the abdominal midline and is separated by the linea alba, which is wider in the upper abdomen and narrower below the umbilicus. The muscle has tendinous intersections, usually three in number: one in the epigastrium, one at the level of the umbilicus, and one between the other two. A fourth intersection, if present, is situated below the umbilicus. The anterior rectus sheath is attached to the muscle at these intersections, whereas the posterior rectus sheath is not. The anterior rectus sheath is present over the muscle along its whole length, but the posterior rectus sheath is absent in the lower part, below the arcuate line. This is the area of potential weakness when the lower rectus myocutaneous flap is used for breast reconstruction.

Arterial Supply

The superior epigastric artery is one of the two terminal branches of the internal mammary artery. It enters the abdominal wall below the seventh costal cartilage and divides into the superficial and deep epigastric systems. The superficial branch supplies the skin and subcutaneous tissue of the upper abdomen up to the level of the umbilicus. This branch communicates with the deep system via intercostal perforators and also by way of vertical rows of perforators through the rectus muscle and the anterior rectus sheath. Such is the arterial supply of the skin and subcutaneous tissue of the upper rectus flap. There are two rows of vertical lines of perforators—one on the medial part and the other on the lateral part of the anterior rectus sheath. The size of the perforators is greater in the periumbilical area. Just above the umbilicus, the deep superior epigastric artery communicates with the terminal branches of the deep inferior epigastric artery through "choke vessels" or arteriolae.[8] The deep superior epigastric artery runs deep at the upper end of the rectus muscle on the medial side of the muscle, between the posterior rectus sheath and the muscle. Here, the pedicle can be visualized and palpated when the muscle is turned over during operation. In the midabdomen, the deep superior epigastric artery is in the middle of the rectus muscle, where it joins with the deep inferior epigastric branches.

Venous Drainage

The veins of the skin and subcutaneous tissue of the upper abdomen are drained along the superficial epigastric vein, which communicates with the deep system via two vertical rows of venous perforators through the anterior rectus sheath. These also communicate with the veins along the intercostal perforators. The veins along the superficial and deep epigastric arteries end at the internal mammary vein. The superficial veins on each side of the midline also communicate with each other.[1]

Nerve Supply

The nerve supply is through the intercostal branches of the seventh, eighth, and ninth lower intercostal nerves. The nerves enter above the posterior rectus sheath at the lateral end of the rectus muscle, then enter it on the middle of its deep surface.[2] Splitting the rectus muscle laterally will denervate the lateral half and cause atrophy and fibrosis. The intercostal nerves convey both motor and sensory impulses.

Patient Selection

Adequate time should be spent during the initial physical examination of the patient. The general health status should be preoperatively evaluated. If the patient had preoperative chemotherapy, blood count and coagulation status should be checked.

During local examination, the status of the chest skin, pectoral muscle, and mastectomy scar are evaluated. The opposite breast is evaluated regarding the shape and size of the tissue. Any infraclavicular hollowness is noted. The abdominal wall is examined regarding shape, adequacy of the soft tissue in the upper abdomen, and presence of any scar or abdominal wall weakness.

Because the upper rectus flap has very good blood supply compared with the lower rectus flap, the former has fewer contraindications. Obesity, chronic smoking, advanced age, and diabetes in well-controlled patients, for example, are not contraindications in upper rectus flap operation. The main contraindications are listed in Table 15.1.

The operation and possible complications should be discussed with the patient in detail preoperatively. Immediate reconstruction following mastectomy can be performed provided good cooperation exists between the general surgeon and the plastic surgeon regarding scheduling time, and as long as the patient had adequate consultation with the plastic surgeon before mastectomy. The patient should not have unrealistic expectations about the result of the operation.

Patient Preparation and Surgical Technique

The patient undergoes medical evaluation 24 to 48 hours prior to operation.

The preoperative flap marking is done on the operating table, immediately before the operation.

Because blood transfusion is not necessary, no preparation for autologous blood transfusion is needed.

An elliptic skin island flap is marked on the upper abdomen. A 10- to 12-cm-wide flap in the center usually is adequate. The upper border of the flap runs at the level of the xiphoid process, whereas the lower border runs just above the umbilicus *(Fig. 15.1)*. The inframammary fold on the reconstructed side is made 1.5 cm lower than the corresponding inframammary line on the normal side. The outline of the rectus muscle is marked on the reconstructed side. The marking procedure is carried out with the patient in the sitting position.

A large elliptic flap of skin and subcutaneous tissue is raised along the preoperative marking lines. Flap raising is performed in the same manner as with the lower rectus flap.[3] The flap on the opposite side is raised first. Starting at the flank and proceeding medially, the flap is raised above the anterior rectus sheath up to the midline. The position of the perforators coming out through the anterior rectus sheath are noted on this side, in order to save them when raising the flap on the opposite side. The flap is then raised on the ipsilateral side, starting at the flank and proceeding medially superficial to the external oblique muscle sheath and up to the lateral border of the rectus muscle. Dissection then proceeds carefully over the anterior rectus sheath for another one quarter of the width of the anterior muscle rectus sheath until the line of perforators is reached.

The anterior rectus sheath is then opened vertically from the costal cartilage to the level of the umbilicus along the line of perforators. The lateral edge of the rectus muscle is freed from the anterior rectus sheath attachment. The ipsilateral rectus muscle is divided just above the level of the umbilicus and above the third tendinous intersection. The deep superior epigastric pedicle is ligated. Then the ipsilateral flap dissection is performed. The whole width of the rectus muscle and medial three fourths of the anterior rectus sheath are dis-

Table 15.1
Main Contraindications

1. Scar in upper abdomen
2. Hernia or weakness in upper abdomen
3. Patient unwilling to accept scar in the midabdomen
4. Inadequate bulk in upper abdominal wall

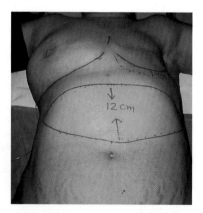

FIG. 15.1

sected, and the rectus muscle is separated from the posterior rectus sheath by gentle fingertip dissection up to the midline and the level of the xiphoid costal cartilage. The rectus muscle is not split laterally for abdominal wall reconstruction, because that would cause denervation of the lateral fibers and damage the venous perforators. The lateral part of the muscle becomes atrophic.[1,2,5] Some attachments of the rectus muscle on the costal cartilages are carefully detached to release tension on the flap pedicle. The eighth intercostal nerve and vessels are also divided to release tension.

After pedicle tension is released, the flap is put back into its original position in the abdomen. Flap vascularity can be ascertained by 10 ml of I.V. fluorescein dye and examined with Wood's light after 8 to 10 minutes. Normally, satisfactory fluorescence is obtained along the whole length of the flap; if any area appears doubtful, it is discarded.

The mastectomy site is now opened by excising the mastectomy scar. A breast pocket of adequate size is made with sharp dissection. The lower part of the pocket is created under the skin and connected with the abdominal wound through a large tunnel. A tunnel of adequate size is necessary to prevent any compression on the flap pedicle. After adequate hemostasis is obtained, the flap is transferred to the breast pocket through the tunnel. The amount of flap skin to be buried underneath the breast pocket is marked and de-epithelialized. The flap is set on the breast pocket by trial and error, until a breast mound of adequate shape is obtained. If necessary, some skin area can be excised in the lower part of the chest wall for better flap placement. The flap pedicle will tolerate some amount of rotation without any problem. Resection of the costal cartilage is never necessary for the flap to reach the chest area. If the flap is very thick with excess subcutaneous fat, some of it can be removed from zone III or IV.[3]

During the abdominal wall closure the operating

Table 15.2
Postoperative Care

1. Early ambulation is encouraged

2. Patient should wear a brassiere for support for 2 weeks when up and about, until the postoperative swelling disappears

3. Gradually increasing activity is encouraged. No strenuous activity is advised for 3 weeks

4. Patients are advised not to start smoking until at least 1 week after the operation

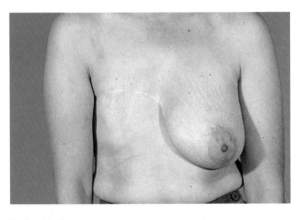

FIG. 15.2

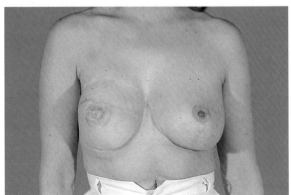

FIG. 15.3

table is flexed. No undermining of the lower abdomen is necessary, and the position of the umbilicus need not be changed. The lateral edge of the anterior rectus sheath is sutured to the linea alba with interrupted sutures. Synthetic mesh can be used to strengthen the repair if necessary, although it is seldom needed. Drains are placed in both chest and abdominal wounds, and brought out separately through stab incisions. Subcutaneous tissues and skin are then closed. Postoperative care is covered in Table 15.2.

Complications

Complications are rare. This flap has very good blood supply, and necrosis is seen very seldom. Because the posterior rectus sheath is stronger in the upper abdomen, the incidence of abdominal wall weakness or hernia is rare.

Seroma, hematoma, wound infection, scar hypertrophy or stretching do occur, but are not common when hemostasis and wound closure are performed carefully.

Reconstruction of the Nipple-Areola Complex

This reconstruction is performed 6 to 8 weeks after the breast mound reconstruction, when the flap has settled down. At this time, the exact site of the new nipple and areola can be determined. This procedure is usually done on an outpatient basis.

Operation on Opposite Breast

Sometimes the opposite breast needs to be altered in shape (e.g., reduction, augmentation, or mastopexy) to obtain symmetry with the reconstructed side. This procedure is carried out at the same time when the nipple-areola complex is reconstructed on the new breast. *Figure 15.2* shows a 39-year-old patient with modified radical mastectomy of the right breast. The left breast has moderate hypertrophy and ptosis. *Figure 15.3* reveals the right breast after upper TRAM flap reconstruction, and the left breast after mastopexy and slight reduction. The 42-year-old woman shown in *Figure 15.4* had a modified radical mastectomy of the right breast before reconstruction with an ipsilateral upper rectus myocutaneous flap. The left breast was operated on for symmetry. Of note, the position of the umbilicus was not altered by the abdominal wound closure *(Fig. 15.5)*.

Discussion

The upper rectus myocutaneous flap is very reliable and stable when used for breast reconstruction following mastectomy. The blood supply and venous drainage of this flap have been extensively studied by several investigators,[1,5,8] and found to be superior to those of the lower rectus flap. Blood transfusion is not necessary with an upper rectus flap operation.

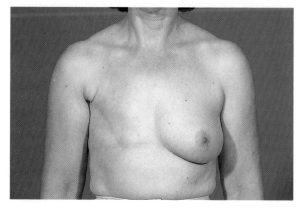

FIG. 15.4

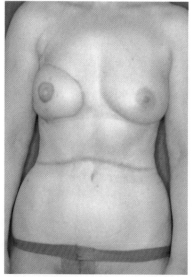

FIG. 15.5

The posterior rectus sheath is stronger in the upper abdomen. Therefore, a repair in the upper abdominal wall remains stronger than in the lower abdomen, and the possibility of hernia is reduced.

The skin of the upper abdomen has better texture. Stretch marks from pregnancy are seen more commonly in the lower than in the upper abdomen. A breast reconstructed from the upper rectus flap has better skin quality and aesthetic appearance.

The operation is easier and quicker when the upper rectus flap is used. Undermining of the lower abdomen is not necessary during abdominal wall closure, which saves time without disturbing the blood supply of the umbilicus and lower abdominal wall. In addition, the lower half of the rectus muscle is spared.

Contrary to common belief, the upper abdominal wall has adequate bulk. Distribution of abdominal wall fat has been studied in cadavers, and it was found that fat is mainly distributed in bulk in the periumbilical area and flanks.[4] This distribution allows more bulk in the upper than in the lower rectus flap. Moreover, because the upper rectus flap can be used almost entirely, it adds more bulk than that obtained with the lower rectus flap.

It is sometimes questioned whether the pedicle length of the upper rectus flap is adequate to avoid tension. No problems were encountered when the ipsilateral flap had been used. Detachment of some rectus muscle fibers from the lower costal cartilages further relieves pedicle tension. In no case, in my experience and the experiences of others,[7] was resection of the cartilage necessary.

The presence of a scar in the midabdomen after using the upper rectus flap has been criticized because it lies in an exposed area, whereas a scar from a lower rectus flap lies hidden in the lower abdomen. This is not a valid criticism because fashions change, and the skin left exposed one year may well be covered during the next one.

REFERENCES

1. Carramenha e Costa MA, Carriquiry C, Vasconez LO, et al: An anatomic study of the venous drainage of the transverse rectus abdominis myocutaneous flap. *Plast Reconstr Surg* 1987;79:208.
2. Duchateau J, Declety A, Lejour M: Innervation of the rectus abdominis muscle: implications for rectus flaps. *Plast Reconstr Surg* 1988; 82:223.
3. Hartrampf CR, Scheflan M, Black PW: Breast reconstruction with a transverse abdominal island flap. *Plast Reconstr Surg* 1982; 69:216.
4. Markman B, Barton FE Jr: Anatomy of the subcutaneous tissue of the trunk and lower extremity. *Plast Reconstr Surg* 1987; 80:248.
5. Moon HK, Taylor GI: The vascular anatomy of rectus abdominis myocutaneous flaps based on the deep superior epigastric system. *Plast Reconstr Surg* 1988; 82:815.
6. Mukherjee RP, Gottlieb V, Hacker LC: Experience with the ipsilateral upper TRAM flap for postmastectomy breast reconstruction. *Ann Plast Surg* 1989; 23:187.
7. Slavin SA, Goldwyn RM: The midabdominal rectus abdominis myocutaneous flap: review of 236 flaps. *Plast Reconstr Surg* 1988; 81:189.
8. Taylor GI, Palmer JH: The vascular territories (angiosomes) of the body: experimental study and clinical applications. *Br J Plast Surg* 1987; 40:113.

CHAPTER·16

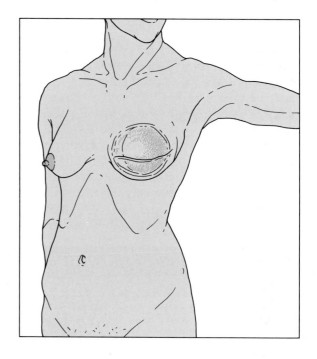

Polyurethane-Covered Implants and Permanent Tissue Expanders for Immediate Reconstruction

Henry C. Vasconez, MD

POLYURETHANE-COVERED IMPLANTS

The smooth wall silicone gel implant *(Fig. 16.1)* was introduced by Cronin and Gerow[4] in 1963. Since then, there have been many variations of this type, including models with softer gels, high silicone crosslinking, thicker shells to prevent silicone leaking, double lumen, and high profile, all in an effort to obtain a more satisfactory result in esthetic augmentation mammaplasties or more adequate projection and ptosis in breast reconstruction.

In the early 1970s, Ashley[1] introduced a polyurethane-covered prosthesis, calling it the "natural Y wide breast prosthesis." Some enthusiasm was generated by this type *(Fig. 16.2)*, and clinical experience was subsequently reported by Capozzi and Pennisi[3] in 1981. Interest increased more recently, after the very detailed reports of Hester et al[5] indicated that the polyurethane-covered prosthesis had just about solved the problem of capsular contracture not only in patients undergoing esthetic augmentation mammaplasty, but also among difficult cases of reconstruction of the breast following modified radical or subcutaneous mastectomy. According to these investigators, the polyurethane-covered prosthesis offers an excellent option to patients with multiply recurring capsular contractures. They suggest replacing the smooth silicone type of implant with a polyurethane-covered one, and inserting it in a "virgin" territory. This means that if the implant had been submuscularly placed, for example, a new plane should be created either subglandularly or subcutaneously. On those occasions when it is not possible to change the plane of reinsertion of the prosthesis, total or subtotal excision of the capsule is advocated.

The most recent introduction in this field has been the textured silicone type of implant *(Fig. 16.3)*, which apparently has a performance similar to those covered with polyurethane. It borrows a similar irregular surface cover to produce the same biochemical effects on the capsule in formation, yet it does not exert the same biochemical effects as the polyurethane-covered prosthesis. However, the experience garnered with textured silicone is not sufficient for a final pronouncement.

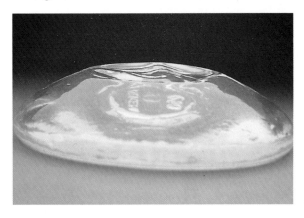

FIG. 16.1

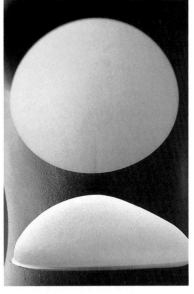

FIG. 16.2

Biologic Considerations

It is important to realize that a comparison of smooth silicone implants and textured or polyurethane-covered ones requires dealing with different biologic processes. After a smooth implant is inserted, passive healing takes place. With a less vascular structure wholly enveloping the implant and contractile forces firmly pulling in unison, capsular contracture occurs *(Fig. 16.4)*. Most times the capsule is quite loose and the result is a freely moving implant. In a large percentage of cases the implant becomes almost imperceptible to the touch, yielding perhaps the nicest type of reconstruction. The unfortunate unpredictability of this excellent result has led a number of plastic surgeons to choose an alternative method that gives more reliable outcomes.

The textured silicone implant has a porous silicone surface with a pore diameter of 300 to 800 microns. Such a surface only allows disorganized tissue ingrowth that does not penetrate the implant. The parallel collagen fibers are stretched, producing tension that impairs vascularity *(Fig. 16.5)*. Preliminary studies indicate no degradation of this textured surface.

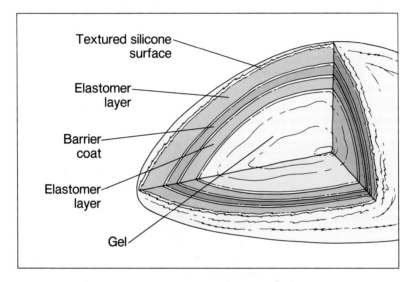

Textured silicone surface
Elastomer layer
Barrier coat
Elastomer layer
Gel

FIG. 16.3

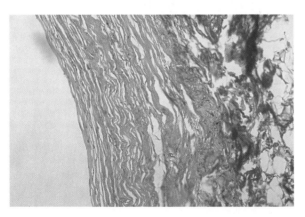

FIG. 16.4 *(Courtesy of Surgitek Medical Engineering Corp.)*

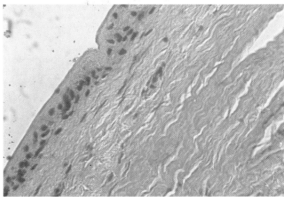

FIG. 16.5 *(Courtesy of Surgitek Medical Engineering Corp.)*

The presently available polyurethane-covered prostheses—either Meme® *(Fig. 16.6)* or Replicon® *(Fig. 16.7)*—are an improved version of the Ashley[1] prosthesis. The polyurethane now used is laser-cut, has a finer foam, and a stronger skeletal base. The result is a biologically more stable material. In addition, the silicone gel is highly cross-linked, which allows shaping for projection and reduces silicone loss. The Meme prosthesis usually is a low profile and wider-based version, whereas the Replicon and the Meme MP have a higher profile and are preferred for reconstructive purposes.

The prevention of spherical capsular contracture by the polyurethane foam coating of mammary implants is said to be due to the textured surface of the polyurethane particles *(Figs. 16.8, 16.9)*. Microtexturing the surface of soft tissue implants tends to disrupt linear capsular contracture formation and increases the vascularity at the soft tissue-implant interface. This vascular, hypercellular response apparently inhibits the ingress of fibroblasts into the capsule by phagocytically active macrophages, and by the prevention of linear contracture around the implant by formation of many microcapsules around the polyurethane particles.

It is not known whether the polyurethane is thoroughly degradable and over what length of time it will do so. Degradation products of polyurethane have been recovered in the urine. One would think that a delayed formation of capsular contracture would ensue after the removal of the periprosthetic tissue. Apparently this does not occur, as stated by Hester et al,[5] who have followed patients for up to 4 years. The longer term 10- and 20-year follow-up studies are as yet unavailable.

Clinical Differences of Smooth and Polyurethane (Textured) Implants

From the clinical standpoint it is important to realize the different biologic reactions to the two implants, particularly as they relate to the location of

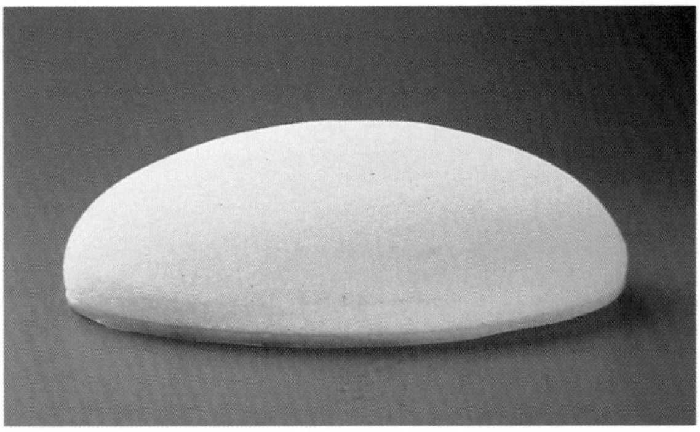

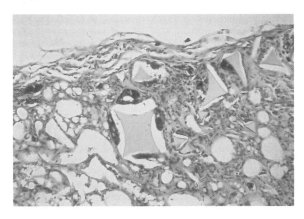

FIG. 16.6 *(Courtesy of Surgitek Medical Engineering Corp.)*

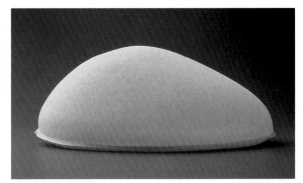

FIG. 16.7 *(Courtesy of Surgitek Medical Engineering Corp.)*

FIG. 16.8 *(Courtesy of Surgitek Medical Engineering Corp.)*

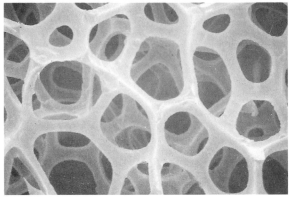

FIG. 16.9 *(Courtesy of Surgitek Medical Engineering Corp.)*

the inframammary fold. If a breast is reconstructed with a smooth implant, some degree of capsular contracture is assumed. Consequently, the pocket is dissected 4 to 5 cm lower than the contralateral normal inframammary fold. Even if the fold turns out to be too low because of a soft capsule, it can subsequently be elevated by taping it or with percutaneous sutures. On the other hand, the assumption with the polyurethane (textured) implant is that it is placed with a multitude of little pins, and that it will remain immobile in the place it is put. Consequently, when a breast is reconstructed with this implant, the location of the inframammary fold is carefully chosen, and its lower edge is determined to be level with or no more than 1 cm lower than the contralateral inframammary fold.

The textured implants have a different feel in the breast than the smooth silicone implants. An excellent result with the smooth gel implant is superior to the predictably constant result of the textured polyurethane-covered implant. Yet it is this predictability which is partly responsible for the re-

cent enthusiasm toward textured implants. Because they remain stationary, surgical techniques have been suggested in an effort to obtain further projection. Specifically, these implants are stacked: a smaller implant is placed on top of a larger implant *(Fig. 16.10.A)* or under it *(Fig. 16.10.B)*. One should remember, however, that projection is determined by the curved distance from the mid sternum to the anterior axillary line. Thus, if there is minimal skin to stretch out, implant stacking will result in tight skin closure with possible exposure of the implant.

Clinical Experience with Implants and Autogenous Tissue

The enormous popularity of the transverse rectus abdominis muscle (TRAM) flap is due to its tremendous versatility in re-creating a new breast. Its other advantages, such as providing an improved abdominal contour and a soft, long-lasting autogenous breast mound, are discussed elsewhere in this book. In recent years, the use of polyurethane-

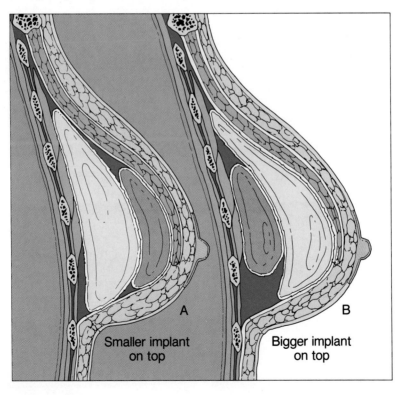

A
Smaller implant
on top

B
Bigger implant
on top

FIG. 16.10

covered implants has helped control the problem of capsular contracture, and their combined use with autogenous tissue also is increasing in popularity. Yet in certain situations, such as a large mastectomy defect or a large contralateral breast, the goal of adequate projection and symmetry is difficult to obtain even with the TRAM flap. In cases of bilateral breast reconstruction the problem is even more enhanced. In such situations, a polyurethane-covered prosthesis placed under the TRAM flap (and often completely covered by it) gives a most satisfactory result. Implants of different size and projection are tried to choose those providing appropriate projection and symmetry.

The implants are preferably placed under the muscle flap to increase tissue ingrowth into the implant surface. Other flaps, such as the latissimus dorsi flap, can be combined with polyurethane-covered prostheses to provide satisfactory results.

Clinical Case

Figures 16.11–16.13 show a 56-year-old patient who underwent modified mastectomy for carcinoma of the breast 3 months earlier. There were no positive nodes, and the patient did not require adjunctive therapy (neither chemotherapy nor endocrine manipulation). She had a well-healed

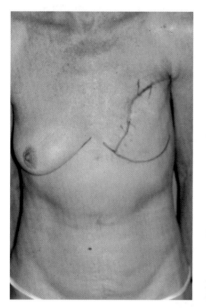
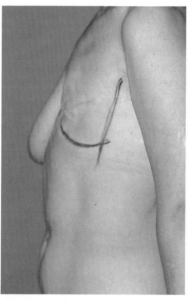
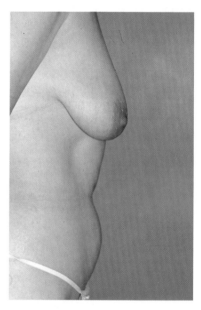

FIG. 16.11   **FIG. 16.12**   **FIG. 16.13**

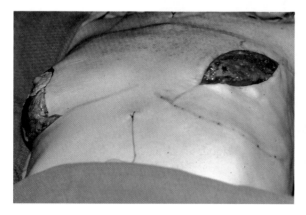
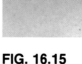

FIG. 16.14   **FIG. 16.15**

oblique scar. The skin was relatively tight, but the pectoralis major muscle was normally innervated. The opposite breast was ptotic, soft, and devoid of any suspicious mass.

Our plan was to reconstruct the left breast by advancing sufficient upper abdominal skin to obtain projection, creating the inframammary fold at the same level or 1 cm below the contralateral one, and inserting a polyurethane-covered prosthesis. In an effort to obtain symmetry, we decided to reduce ptosis on the right breast by inserting a smaller polyurethane-covered prosthesis.

Figure 16.14 shows the open mastectomy scar, the dissection underneath the pectoralis major muscle superiorly, and the subcutaneous dissection down to the costal margin inferiorly.

In *Figure 16.15,* the incision line indicates the level of the inframammary fold.

Figure 16.16 outlines the planned ptosis correction and augmentation mammaplasty for the right breast. A portion of the skin has been de-epithelialized to decrease the skin envelope.

Figure 16.17 shows the sizer for the polyurethane-type implants (Replicon type).

After the sizer prosthesis was inserted underneath the pectoralis major muscle on both sides *(Fig. 16.18),* the patient was moved to a sitting position to check for symmetry. Because of lack of skin, we accepted a slightly diminished projection on the left side. We did not think that it would be safe to stack implants because, as mentioned earlier, lack of skin is a limiting factor.

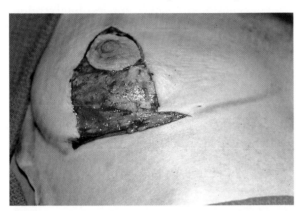

FIG. 16.16

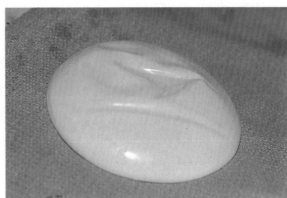

FIG. 16.17

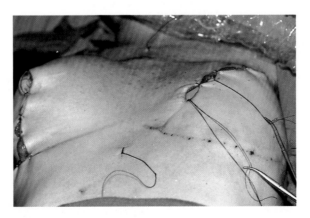

FIG. 16.18

Figures 16.19 and *16.20* show the method of insertion of the polyurethane-covered prosthesis. Because disruption of the polyurethane coating must be avoided, the prosthesis is inserted through a cellophane bag that is twisted distally. To facilitate the insertion, we suggest making a slightly larger incision.

Figure 16.21 shows the breast reconstruction after we placed the permanent polyurethane implants. Note that on the left side the prosthesis is only partially covered by the pectoralis major muscle. Also note the percutaneous creation of the inframammary fold by approximation of the subcutaneous tissue to the intercostal spaces on the left side.

The patient is shown immediately at the end of the procedure in *Figure 16.22*.

PERMANENT TISSUE EXPANDER (BECKER PROSTHESIS)

An attractive concept in reconstruction of the breast has been introduced by Becker,[2] with his ingenious design of a permanent expander prosthesis *(Fig. 16.23)*. The Becker model comprises a silicone gel shell encapsulating a saline nucleus of variable volume. The prosthesis has an inflation portal through which it can be percutaneously inflated to a desired level. When proper size and volume have been obtained, the portal may be removed under local anesthesia through a small incision. Thus, the implant is left in place and a second, larger operative procedure is avoided. This method therefore brings together the advantages of tissue expansion and single surgical intervention.

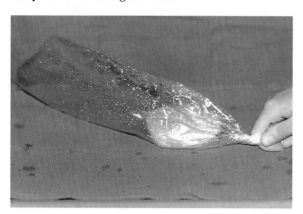

FIG. 16.19

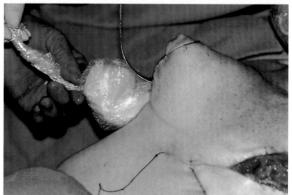

FIG. 16.20

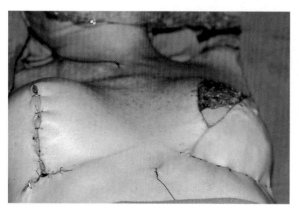

FIG. 16.21

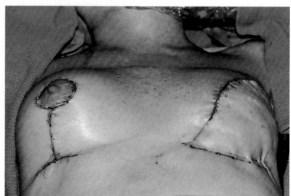

FIG. 16.22

In addition, by varying the inflated volumes, the surgeon may attempt to achieve satisfactory symmetry with the opposite breast. The Becker prosthesis would be particularly useful in bilateral reconstruction, when mastectomies of different type or different amounts of skin have been removed and prostheses of different size are necessary.

However, the disadvantages are considerable and should be kept in mind when choosing this method of reconstruction. First, the Becker prosthesis takes away the main advantage of tissue expansion, that is, the preparation of the patient for a second operative procedure in which asymmetry associated with the position of the implant, volume, or severe capsular contracture can be corrected.

Second, the initial placement of the Becker implant is critical, because any slight discrepancy in pocket size or implant position will be evident during the expansion process and will require correction if symmetry is to be obtained.

Third, there is a limit to the expansion that can be obtained with these implants. Although it is true that one can overinflate, as was done in our illustrative patient, the versatility of injection volume is limited.

Finally, removal of the remote reservoir is rather difficult if it is done under local anesthesia, and may be accompanied by inadvertent rupture of the implant and silicone leakage.

Regardless of the disadvantages, the concept is sound. Perhaps further experience with this method will increase its reliability and provide more predictable results.

The following case reveals some of the problems encountered with the Becker prosthesis.

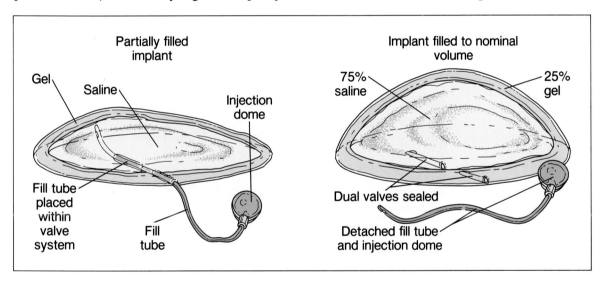

FIG. 16.23

Clinical Case

The patient shown preoperatively in *Figures 16.24–16.26* is a 40-year-old woman with a long history of bilateral fibrocystic disease, whose left breast biopsy showed lobular carcinoma in situ. She also had a very strong family history of breast cancer—her mother and maternal aunt had developed the disease at premenopausal ages.

Bilateral mastectomies were carried out through transverse incisions. Ellipses of skin which included the nipple were removed, followed by axillary dissections. The pathology report of the respective specimens showed lobular carcinoma in two sites, with proliferative fibrocystic disease in the left breast and proliferative fibrocystic disease with atypical lobular hyperplasia in the right breast. The lymph node dissection was negative in both breasts.

Figure 16.27 shows the patient in the operating room. The inframammary folds and the skin ellipses to be excised were marked symmetrically on both sides with the patient in the sitting position.

The defects following the bilateral mastectomies are shown in *Figure 16.28*. Becker-type permanent tissue expanders with a nominal implant size of 400 cc were used, one on each side. *Figure 16.29* shows the Becker prosthesis inserted underneath the pectoralis and serratus muscles. The implant at this moment has only 100 cc of gel surrounding an empty nucleus. Note that the injection tube-portal is brought out through a small opening in the serratus muscle; it will be buried subcutaneously at the axillary line. The implant should be filled intraoperatively to a volume that should not exceed one third of the nominal implant size. We injected 100 cc of saline at the end of the operative procedure. Then, over a period of 6 months, the implants were overexpanded with 350 cc of saline for a total volume of 550 cc (100 cc of gel + 100 cc of saline + 350 cc of saline).

Six months after the insertion of the skin expanders, some asymmetry can be seen on both breasts *(Fig. 16.30)*. The right side is laterally displaced and appears to have less projection than the left side. The size of each implant was adjusted at 6

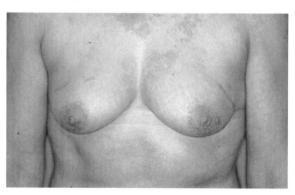

FIG. 16.24

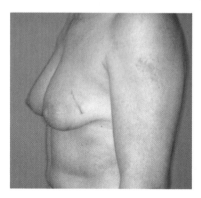

FIG. 16.25

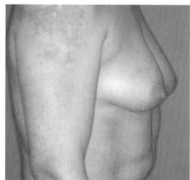

FIG. 16.26

months postop within the recommended volume range. In this case, we withdrew 50 cc of saline to obtain a final total volume of 500 cc.

Figure 16.31 shows the patient prior to the next operative procedure, which involved reconstruction of the nipples and an open capsulotomy on the right breast in an attempt to obtain symmetry.

Completion of the nipple reconstruction with the Skate Method is illustrated in *Figure 16.32.* The patient underwent a Z-plasty on the medial aspect of the right breast. The open capsulotomy (superiorly, inferiorly, and medially) was performed by reopening the lateral portion of the transverse incision.

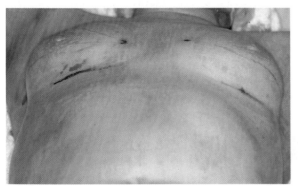

FIG. 16.27

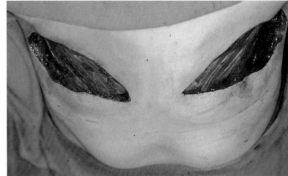

FIG. 16.28

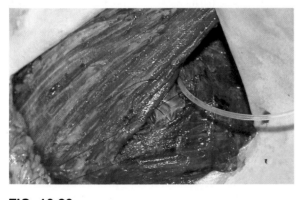

FIG. 16.29

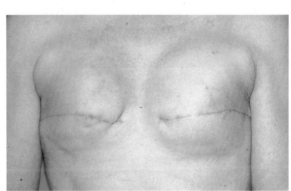

FIG. 16.30

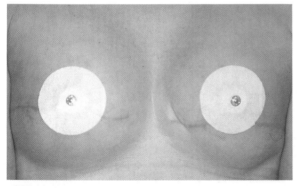

FIG. 16.31

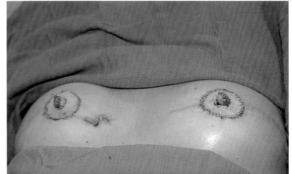

FIG. 16.32

The results, 6 weeks following nipple reconstruction and 7.5 months after the mastectomy with immediate reconstruction, are shown in *Figures 16.33–16.35*. There is still breast asymmetry, with a tighter capsular contraction on the right breast responsible for the downward and medially looking nipple.

Another operation would be required to try to correct the asymmetry, although without any assurance of success.

REFERENCES

1. Ashley FL: A new type of breast prosthesis. *Plast Reconstr Surg 1970;45:421.*

2. Becker H: Breast reconstruction using an inflatable breast implant with detachable reservoir. *Plast Reconstr Surg 1984;73:678.*

3. Capozzi A, Pennisi VR: Clinical experience with polyurethane-covered gel-filled mammary prostheses. *Plast Reconstr Surg 1981;68:512.*

4. Cronin TD, Gerow FJ: Augmentation mammaplasty: a new "natural feel" prosthesis. *Int Congr Ser 1964;66:41.*

5. Hester TR, Nahai F, Bostwick J, Cukic J: A 5-year experience with polyurethane-covered mammary prostheses for treatment of capsular contracture, primary augmentation mammoplasty, and breast reconstruction. *Clin Plast Surg 1988;15(4):569.*

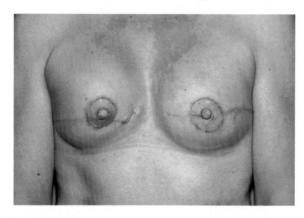

FIG. 16.33

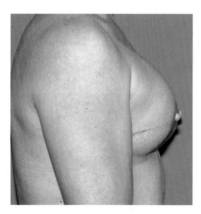

FIG. 16.34

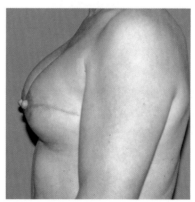

FIG. 16.35